MW01064632

Advance Praise for
Sensory Parenting

I love this book! This is a treasure trove of smart advice for both new and seasoned parents who want to help their newborns, toddlers, and preschoolers feel calm and comfortable in an overstimulating world. Written in a warm, wise, and friendly voice by a parent and occupational therapist team, this book is jam-packed with a comprehensive range of practical suggestions, from mealtime and bedtime to motor milestones and developmentally appropriate toys. It's a must-have resource for parents and early childhood professionals!

LINDSEY BIEL, OTR/L
Coauthor of *Raising a Sensory Smart Child: The Definitive Handbook for Helping Your Child with Sensory Processing Issues*

A useful and accessible tool for both parents and practitioners. I am thrilled to have a resource to recommend to parents about this area of development, which is frequently overlooked or misunderstood. Few, if any, parenting books offer this many tools, tips, and techniques aimed at helping parents nurture and manage aspects of sensory development in children.

BRIAN W. TEMPLE MD, FAAP
Pediatrician in Salem Oregon

Sensory Parenting
From Newborns to Toddlers

PARENTING IS EASIER WHEN YOUR CHILD'S SENSES ARE HAPPY!

BRITT COLLINS, MS, OTR/L
and JACKIE LINDER OLSON

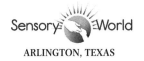

SENSORY PARENTING: Newborns to Toddlers

All marketing and publishing rights guaranteed to and reserved by:

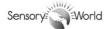

A proud imprint of Future Horizons

721 W. Abram Street
Arlington, Texas 76013
800-489-0727
817-277-0727
817-277-2270 (fax)
E-mail: *info@sensoryworld.com*
www.sensoryworld.com

© 2010 Britt Collins, MS, OTR/L, & Jackie Linder Olson

Book design © TLC Graphics, *www.TLCGraphics.com*
Cover by Monica Thomas; Interior by Erin Stark

Cover photo: ©iStockphoto.com/Mike Grindley

All rights reserved.

Printed in the United States of America

No part of this book may be reproduced in any manner whatsoever without written permission of Future Horizons, Inc., except in the case of brief quotations embodied in reviews.

ISBN: 9781935567226

For Odin and Mary Allison

Table of Contents

Foreword..ix

Preface..xiii

Acknowledgments xvii

Introduction to the Seven Senses.....................................xix

Chapter 1: Preparing for Baby 1
  A Sensory-Friendly Nursery..3
  Organizing Your Home...11
  Vaccines...16

Chapter 2: Your Newborn (0-6 Months)........................19
  Bonding with Your Baby 19
  Bathing, Changing Diapers, Dressing, and Swaddling............25
  Baby in Motion..31
  Feeding Your Baby 35
  Sleeping...42
  The Importance of Tummy Time......................................49
  Play 51
  Developmental Milestones, 0 to 6 Months 55

Chapter 3: Baby Life (6 Months to 1 Year)......................59
  Rolling Over, Sitting Up, and Reaching..............................59
  Crawling—Motor Planning...61
  Activities and Technology...62
  Teaching Your Baby Sign Language 69

Play 70

Developmental Milestones, 6 Months to 1 Year 74

Chapter 4: Toddler Time (1 to 2 Years) 77

Baby Learns to Walk 77

Baby's Sensory Systems 81

Sleep Cycles Change 90

Play 92

Developmental Milestones, 1 to 2 Years 96

Chapter 5: Baby's Caregivers 103

Babysitters, Nannies, and Daycare 103

Siblings and Other Family Members 113

Pets 115

Stay-at-Home Mom (or Dad!) 122

Mommy Goes to Work (Pumping, Guilt, and Alone Time) 126

Chapter 6: Growing Up (2 to 3 Years) 131

Your Not-So-Terrible 2-Year-Old 131

Communicating with Your Child 138

Choices: My Way or My Way 142

Potty Training 144

Toddler Hygiene 152

Your Toddler Sleeps 158

Social Skills 161

Tantrums, Discipline, Redirecting, and Prevention 165

Outings 172

Play 185

Developmental Milestones, 2 to 3 Years 197

Chapter 7: Evaluating Your Child's Senses 201

Is Your Child Hyper- or Hyposensitive? 201

Will He/She Grow Out of It? What If I Ignore It? 205

Occupational Therapy and Sensory Integration 205

Does My Child Have SPD, Autism, or ADHD? 210

Auditory Processing Disorder 223

Chapter 8: Therapies for the Senses 227
The Mouth 227
The Eyes: Light Therapy 233
The Nose: Aromatherapy 234
Music Therapy 236
The Ears 242
The Skin: Baby Massage 246
Acupressure 248

Chapter 9: Environmental Factors 251
Toxins in Your Home 251
Diet 257
Food Allergies and Intolerances 264

Chapter 10: Medical Concerns 271
Preemies 271
Hospital Stays 277
Cerebral Palsy, Hypotonia, Mental Retardation, and Seizures ... 282

Epilogue 285

Appendix A: Parent Survey 287

Appendix B: Must-Have Baby Kit 303

References 305

Resources 307

Index 311

About the Authors 319

Foreword

"In this life we cannot do great things.
We can only do small things with great love."

MOTHER TERESA

WITH GREAT JOY I UNFOLDED THE PAGES OF *SENSORY PARENTING*, BY BRITT Collins and Jackie Olson. As I read, I felt that they were talking to me about my first baby, my little one going from a newborn to an infant, an infant to a toddler, and a toddler to a preschooler.

For parents who have young children with sensory challenges, this is an amazing book. It is honest but funny, self-reflective and instructive. I love the way all parenting styles are considered and accepted. The parent's right to choose is highlighted, and the book does not preach the *right* way versus the wrong way. It maintains the principle that children and families are different; what is right for one family may not be the best practice for another family.

This book is a combination of a how-to manual and an insightful journey into the world of newborns, infants, toddlers, and preschoolers. The voice of the book is clear and convincing, genuine and positive. The information is "help," but the message is "hope." While the ideas for taking care of your little one are extremely practical and important, the message of taking care of yourself and understanding the needs of your child are paramount. I love that about this book. Love is the top consideration, and techniques and suggestions are about making life for the parents and child easier and more comfortable, and more about the relationship they share.

Most books about sensory processing and sensory-processing challenges read more like recipes than prose. But *Sensory Parenting* is intuitive, honest, and engaging. "Help—there's a hot-pink Hello Kitty about to attack me!" say Collins and Olson, when they discuss how to build a sensory-friendly nursery. "I'm the first to admit I love to blare music while I drive," they confess, when discussing the introduction of auditory stimulation into a baby's world.

The tips for where to obtain items are excellent, with dozens of Web site references to obtain special equipment and materials. The focus is on low-cost, natural products that most could afford, not on specialized therapy equipment. Dealing with issues from vaccines to nursing, learning second languages, Gymboree, and choosing nannies and daycare, Collins and Olson offer advice that is common sense yet based on a foundation of developmental and behavioral expertise.

I think you will love the lists of developmentally appropriate toys at each age and the normal developmental milestones listed for each age group. The red flags, or "things to look out for" at each stage of development, are short and pragmatic and will help new parents and professionals alike to stay tuned to development at every age and stage. Not only will you love them, but you will also use them! I know I would!

Jackie, with her "Mom Tips," and Britt, with her "Occupational Therapist Tips," have created a partnership that mirrors the partnership occupational therapists should build with parents of infants, toddlers, and preschool children who have special sensory needs. In fact, this is a great book for parents of all children, because all children have sensory needs, either respected or not noticed.

On going back to work, "What to do? Who am I again?" is especially poignant for those of us who do have careers. Every working parent's worst fear comes out at that time—as well as stress, doubt, exhaustion, and individual differences. There is no preaching in this book, just an acceptance of choices and options and a theme of attending to the sensory needs of all—the child, his or her siblings, and yourself. This book would make an exceptional gift to anyone who is expecting a baby or who has a young child, from a newborn to a toddler.

In the last few sections of this book, more technical issues like the types of Sensory Processing Disorder, therapies for the senses, environmental factors, and medical concerns are tackled. While each of the subjects is worth its own book rather than a chapter, Olson and Collins have done a nice job of summarizing complicated material in a way that will be understandable to parents and useful to professionals. While not all of the suggestions have an evidence-based (research) approach, I admire the direct manner in which the material has been gathered and presented.

They close with, "It's never too late to start becoming more aware of your own senses and those of your family members." I couldn't agree more!

And I close with a thank-you to Britt and Jackie for their hard work and their great contribution to the growing literature in the field of Sensory Processing Disorder.

Bravo!

LUCY JANE MILLER
Director of STAR (Sensory Therapies And Research) Center and
Executive Director of the Sensory Processing Disorder Foundation
Greenwood Village, Colorado
July 23, 2010

Preface

THE WORLD SEEMS LIKE IT'S SPINNING AT A FASTER PACE THESE DAYS, AND we are constantly inundated with sensory information. The bright light from the computer screen, flashing billboards, phones ringing, televisions yammering—it can be overwhelming for adults, but think about it from a baby or a child's point of view. The world can be a wonderful and exciting place, but it can also be a loud, scary, and physically painful one, especially if a child's sensory-processing systems are a little off—if his or her eyes, ears, and other sensory systems are not protected and properly guided.

As an occupational therapist (Britt) and mom (Jackie) team, we have compiled helpful tips and guidelines in looking at the world through your child's sensory systems. Sometimes a tantrum isn't just about the cookie he wants. It could be that the sun is in his eyes, and the noise of the outdoor concert has deregulated his auditory processing. We help you look at your parenting skills and the choices you make by taking into consideration cues and behaviors from your children's internal and external symptoms.

We believe that all parents want their kids to be happy. In addition, we all want our kids to live productive and fulfilling lives. One way to help them is to make sure they're processing at their highest capability. We're living in an exciting time, a time of extraordinary technology and vast progress, but also a time in which people are open to new ideas and sharing more emotional data than ever before. Babies and toddlers don't have the language to articulate what they're feeling. As parents, we must realize that all this information can be stressful and draining, so we'd like to help sift through the overload and be the voice of the senses.

One of the many responsibilities of occupational therapists is to teach life skills: dressing, brushing teeth, eating, playing, and going to school. Occupational therapists help children with social skills, motor coordination skills, and fine-, visual-, and gross-motor skills, along with how to process the various types of sensory information that is coming into our bodies every minute of the day. One example of this could be sitting at home, enjoying a nice, relaxing book while the washing machine runs in the background. For some people, this is a nice hum that does not distract them from their book—but for others, the sound is excruciating and prevents them from focusing on the book they are reading. Looking at this from a child's perspective, think about what a child with sensitivities to light and sound might experience in a grocery store. Do you wonder why you see a child having a tantrum in the aisle of the store? Maybe she really wants that bag of chips, but maybe she is so overwhelmed by the situation, she can only scream and cry to drown everything else out.

Play is a huge part of development, and as a parent-therapist team, we encourage parents to incorporate play into their child's daily activities. Various "play" activities may include movement and engagement, which are important for development. Children need to have some sort of structure in their lives, but they also need to understand the importance of self, creativity, connection with others, and survival. Encouraging children to play with educational toys can help increase their attention skills and assist with problem solving and taking an intellectual approach to situations. Movement types of play, such as playing games or sports outside or romping around on a playground, help a child to regulate his or her sensory system and strengthen balance, coordination, and other gross-motor skills. Group-play activities enable the development of social skills and provide an understanding about friendships, winning, and losing, as well as appropriate behaviors.

PREFACE

We created this book to be compatible with other parenting books and many different parenting styles by focusing primarily on a child's senses, both fully functioning systems and those that are considered dysfunctional. We will list options, alternatives, and points to consider, but you'll find that we encourage you to use whatever works best for your family.

Not only will we be talking about your child's sensory systems, but we will encourage you to explore your own, as well. We all have our own sensory sensitivities to some extent—some more than others—and we often become more aware of a sensitivity or dysfunction once we have children. You may become more aware of sounds that bother you or tastes that you've been avoiding for years. Perhaps you realize that you stay away from crowds or that playdates aren't your cup of tea! Don't worry, we're here to try and help pave the sensory road for you and your family.

Note: To make reading easy for you and to keep our message consistent, we will speak to you as one voice. When talking about being a mother, it's written from Jackie's point of view. Britt's voice will come as the occupational-therapist perspective. Both will be referred to as "I."

Acknowledgments

Britt's Acknowledgments

FIRST AND FOREMOST, I WANT TO THANK MY ROCK AND #1 SUPPORTER, Linds. You have always been there for me through this whole process and have brought me such joy in life. Thank you for being so patient with me and for always loving me, no matter what. I also want to thank my family for always believing in me and listening to my crazy dreams in life. If it were not for my sister, I would never have become an occupational therapist, for which I am continuously grateful, as I truly love what I do. Thank you to my friends, who have also been a great support through this writing process, as it has been fun, exciting, and exhausting. Last but not least, thank you Jackie—you have been such an amazing business partner, mom, friend, and supporter! If not for you, I don't know how I would have gotten as far as we've come. Thank you for your endless support and for always believing in me.

Jackie's Acknowledgments

To Kare Bear, for your endless help and friendship. Without you, I would not be able to slay dragons and move mountains or chase rainbows.

To Ekim Rednil, for always believing in me and my dreams, for repeaters, the gift of gab, ten-point-toss-up, and for always taking my any-hour-of-the-night calls.

To Bryce, for paving our own road when the world was against us and for holding my hand through life.

To Julie, for singing to me at night when I was scared, for taking me to Mexico for the first time, for giving me the book on breastfeeding, and for countless other reasons why ILMS.

To Amy, for your honesty and friendship—you set the bar. Meow.

To Hot Nanny, for being more than a business partner, you're a dear friend. You shine when you're working with your kids, and you were truly meant to be an occupational therapist. I'm forever grateful.

To Odin, you own my heart. Everything I do is for you.

From Both of Us

Together we would like to thank our friends and colleagues, who have helped us with this amazing book along the way. Thank you Angie H., Lindsey B., Aviva W., Lucy M., Carol K., Emily S., Shanna M., Jess A., Nicole C., Jen D., Naomi A., Jen H., Khymberleigh, Yamile J., Andy T., Teri A., Andrea L., and Melissa E.

Thank you to all the parents of the babies and children's photos that grace our pages and make us smile.

A very special thank-you to the Future Horizons and Sensory World team: Wayne, Jennifer, Heather, and Erin—we are eternally grateful for this opportunity and to now be a part of your work family. We look forward to a bright future together!

Introduction
to the Seven Senses

THE FIVE SENSES THAT EVERYONE KNOWS ABOUT ARE TASTE, TOUCH, SIGHT, sound, and smell. Each of us also has two additional senses—the vestibular sense and the proprioceptive sense.

Taste originates in the mouth and in the ability to detect flavors. Babies are oral learners, and they will put everything in their mouths, starting at only a few months of age. This helps them learn about their environment. This sense can end up being very important to your baby, especially if she has difficulty trying new foods or flavors when she begins eating.

Touch originates in the skin, which performs a variety of functions and protects the body against injury, infection, and water loss. Your skin helps regulate your body temperature by releasing sweat as needed. It is your largest organ, and your body processes many sensations throughout the skin, such as temperature (hot or cold), texture (smooth or rough), the size of objects, pain, and sensations of pleasure, like being tickled. Many adults and children who have sensory difficulties with touch can be sensitive to tags in their clothes, or they don't like touching gooey things. Your baby may be irritated by certain clothing or the feel of a particular bottle nipple.

Sight is such an amazing sense, and sometimes we take it for granted. The eyes are truly our "windows" to the world. When a baby is born, his sight is limited—he can only see black, white, and shades of gray. One week after birth, however, he begins to see red, yellow, green, and orange. Don't be worried if your baby doesn't immediately focus on your face—this will come with time.

Sound is a complex sense, involving anything we can hear. The auditory system consists of the ears and the brain working together to process frequencies and vibrations into a comprehensible sound. Many babies have auditory issues due to ear infections, but most children will grow out of these sensitivities with proper guidance and assistance.

Your olfactory sense is your sense of *smell.* It is the detection and perception of chemicals coming into the nose and how your brain processes what the smell is. Smell is deeply associated with memory and is the only sense that goes directly to the emotional center of the brain.

The *vestibular* sense is the sense of movement, which governs your balance. It is driven by the fluid in your inner ear and tells us whether our heads are right-side up or upside-down. The vestibular sense also tells us how fast we are moving and whether we are going forward or backward. Someone who has difficulties with vestibular processing may get carsick easily, or a child may like to spin because he seeks more vestibular input to this system.

The *proprioceptive* sense is the input to the muscles and joints that tells us about movement and body position. It tells us where each body part is in relation to another. A child who has difficulties with proprioceptive processing may push so hard on a crayon that it breaks when she is coloring, or she may not be able to close her eyes and touch her nose.

All of these senses work together in what is called *sensory integration and regulation.* Our brains are constantly decoding and processing the information sent by each of these sensory systems simultaneously so that we may understand our world. If one or all of these systems are not functioning properly, you may see changes or struggles in your child. We are here to help you provide a healthy sensory environment for you and your family.

CHAPTER ONE

Preparing for Baby

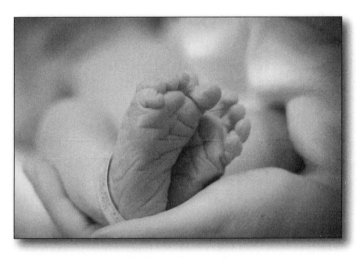

So little and so perfect.
JACKSON, ONE DAY OLD

YOU'VE BEEN PREGNANT FOR A WHILE NOW AND HAVE PROBABLY FELT THE baby kick and move. You've begun researching what to do with your baby and how to take care of him or her. Many new parents and even parents who are going through this for the second or third time forget the little things about the ins and outs of having a newborn in the house. This particular book will take you on a journey of parenting from a sensory perspective.

When preparing for your new arrival, you want to take into consideration the baby's immediate environment—your home. Where will the baby be spending most of his time when he first comes home? Probably with you! What is your house like? Are there other children? Animals? Bright lights, loud noises, strong smells? While your baby is in your belly, he is getting used to the environment that you live in. He hears your voice and the voices of other family members. He gets used to your daily activities. When you are sleeping, he tends to sleep in your belly. When you are active, he tends to be more active. He has learned to regulate himself according to how you have regulated yourself on a daily basis. Once the baby is born, he still maintains some of this regulation from you, but it is very different than swimming in a warm, cozy environment, like he has for the past 9 months!

Wow! He is such a tiny person in such a large world! You really want to make sure he has a suitable environment in which to grow up. Dim the lights a bit, talk in calming voices, and be aware that his auditory system is getting used to the sounds around him. He needs to be snuggled up tight, so be ready to swaddle him to give him a sense of boundaries and some comforting, deep pressure. Keep things simple in the beginning, and as your baby grows and learns, you can add more toys, colors, and sounds to his environment. Allow your newborn to adjust to his new environment as you get the hang of being a new parent! Congratulations, you are about to begin an amazing journey of becoming a parent, and it is an irreversible experience that you will treasure forever. It will not always be easy, but it will ALWAYS be worth it!

As every adult is different, so is every baby. You will quickly learn your baby's temperament and unique behaviors. Some babies are easy, happy, and eager to take on the world, while others may be cranky and uncomfortable and want to hide in their mothers' arms. You may be surprised or disappointed if your baby is tense, sensitive, difficult, or fussy, but remember that comforting your baby may help her grow into a more jovial baby in time. Be compassionate with your baby, and you two will bond and bring out the best in one another.

A Sensory-Friendly Nursery

Visual Considerations

"Help—there's a hot-pink Hello Kitty about to attack me!" The baby's room should be soothing and calming. Save the bright and hectic patterns for the playroom. You want your baby's room to be calming and "Zen-like." As you decorate, think about providing the best, most comfortable environment in which your child will sleep. While your baby is young, she is not going to be in her room much, unless she is sleeping—so don't worry about surrounding her with toys, stuffed animals, or bright colors until she is a little older.

Think about painting the walls of the baby's room a soft and calming color. Blue is reminiscent of water and is cool and promotes relaxation. Green is indicative of nature, which may also be soothing. If you want to add warmth, choose a deeper, darker blue. Use turquoise to create a more "girly" feel to your baby's room, while staying within a tranquil color palate. Or, we also recommend violet for your little one, which is a peaceful color variation. You can accent with reds and yellows, but keep in mind that those colors can be overpowering—especially to a sensory-sensitive child.

Please use nontoxic paint when painting your child's room, which is often labeled "Non-VOC" (volatile organic compounds) or "Zero VOC." Do yourself a favor—buy low-odor paint, as well.

When decorating, try not to clutter the room with a lot of things. Stick to the basics. You need a crib, a changing table with space to put clothes and diapers, and possibly a rocking chair so you can rock your baby to sleep. As your baby gets older, you can begin to add more things to his room, such as toys, pictures on the walls, and other furniture, if needed.

It is helpful for some babies to have a mobile over their beds to help them fall asleep, or, when they wake up, to have something to look at and then hopefully fall back asleep.

Sounds

As someone with auditory issues myself, noises really bother me. I hear everything—the birds chirping, my husband's TV in the other room, and the clock ticking in the hall. It's not a surprise that my son has auditory issues, as well. To help us both sleep, we have an air purifier in our bedroom that hums at night. I figure the air purifier is doing double-duty: The fan provides us with the white noise, while we also benefit from clean air. If we travel, we have to keep the fan on in our hotel room or bring along a small white-noise machine; otherwise, my son and I lie awake, listening to the cars zoom by, bakery trucks delivering bread to the hotel restaurant, and any birds chirping in the vicinity.

If you have other children or a lot of activity going on in your house, be considerate of your baby's sleep cycles. I know many parents who assume that their baby can be trained to sleep while they run the vacuum cleaner and while the chaos of a busy household unfolds, but a baby with sensory processing disorder (SPD) cannot. Using a blender to make a smoothie sends my son into hysterics. He will scream louder than the machine or whatever noise is hurting him. Many children who are sensitive to sounds want to figure out a way to either make it stop or drown it out, just as we do as adults.

As a child, you are most likely going to be unable to make the uncomfortable noise stop, so you begin to cry, scream, or sing really loudly. This helps to cover up the noise that is making you uncomfortable. As a parent, however, we may not understand in the beginning why our child is doing any of these things. You have to take a step back and look at the whole picture and try to figure out why your child is upset.

Slowly introduce your baby to certain noises that she will eventually need to learn to tolerate, but remember that it is okay for you to help regulate your child's sensory system by providing her with a quiet, calming environment. Later on, we will talk more about how to help desensitize your child to certain sensory inputs that help her function in the day-to-day world.

I really enjoy using the womb-sounds bear (a bear with a heartbeat in it, which can be purchased at stores like Target or on *amazon.com*).

If you tie it around the outside of the crib, when your baby awakes in the night and cries, it activates sounds from the womb to help calm her and put her back to sleep. I have had many families provide positive feedback about this particular toy. Some of the womb-sounds bears also play additional calming sounds, and when the child gets older, you can take the noise box out of the bear so she has a soft teddy bear as a toy.

Baby Music

Another thing to think about, if you don't have something like the womb-sounds bear, is music. Some families choose to have soft music playing in the background while their child sleeps; others want their child to learn how to fall asleep in a quiet environment or be able to tolerate sleeping through outside noise, such as the sound of siblings running around downstairs. Each child is different, and you need to accommodate your child's needs, especially in the beginning. A child with SPD may not be able to tolerate even the softest classical music in the background, even though it is supposed to be calming. You need to figure out what works best for your child and then help him slowly adapt to other situations, as well, as he grows and learns to tolerate various sensory inputs from his environment.

Music and memorization go hand in hand. Think about it. People say all the time that they have a horrible memory, but then they can sing along with every song on the radio. Music is often used as a mnemonic device for students who are studying for exams. They may turn their studies into a song to impress it into their memories.

When choosing music for the nursery, here are a few things to keep in mind. If you play stimulating music while your baby is trying to sleep, you'll have an exhausted, wide-awake baby. Music is big business, and producers know that parents want the best music for their babies. With today's technology, it's easy to sample a variety of baby music and purchase the songs you enjoy before the baby arrives.

Studies have also shown that music we listen to while our brains are developing stays with us forever. When I first read this, I thought back to my first musical memories. I can easily recall my first dance-recital song in kindergarten and dancing around my living room while my mother blasted Donna Summers and Abba. I've always had a strong affection for the song "Greensleeves," as well. I asked my parents about this and was told that my mother often played "Greensleeves" on the piano when I was a baby. To this day, that song moves me to my emotional core. So, pick out your baby's first music with that in mind. It's an imprint that you will leave forever.

You must be your baby's acoustical engineer, meaning that you'll need to provide noise control by reducing unwanted sounds and choose which source of music best suits your baby's room. While you will most likely not redesign the baby's room with soundproof walls, you will be in charge of selecting the baby's sound system. Will your baby listen to music on your iPod through speakers? Make sure there is no static while the iPod is idle or in between songs. Will she have her own Barbie CD player? Make sure you don't have a patchy radio signal and that the speakers don't make extra static noises or feedback.

White Noise for Baby

If you are concerned about the street noise outside your home or your neighbor's rowdy weekend parties, you can drown these noises out with white noise. Tranquil noisemakers include options for listening to a babbling brook, dolphins, or a heartbeat. They also have therapeutic sound programs to gently lull baby to sleep. You can find them at retailers such as *www.Brookstone.com.*

The theory behind white noise is that it's a consistent noise that masks other potentially offensive or distracting sounds. Some people find it hard to sleep when it's too quiet or can't sleep while a TV is on, while cars are driving by, or while the icemaker drops ice into a bin every 4 hours. The white noise drowns out other noises so that the brain can relax into sleep mode.

Why would you want your baby to become reliant on white noise to sleep? While we don't want your baby to be reliant on a manmade product, if your baby can't sleep in your home, because of noisy neighbors, barking dogs, or other offensive noises, you'll want her to get peaceful rest. Not all babies need white noise. Some babies can sleep through anything. Parents can vacuum under their cribs, and it doesn't stir the baby. A friend of mine recently had a baby who remained in the hospital for a few months after birth, and now that she's home, her baby needs to have the TV on to fall asleep. During his first few months, the hospital was hectic and noisy and the TV was often on, and that is what he got used to.

Baby Tunes—What to Pick?

There is a wide variety of baby music to choose from. You can easily pick music that will be pleasing for both you and your baby. Classical music is a favorite amongst most parents and can be found in most baby stores, as well as online. While we don't buy into the hype that classical music will make your baby a genius, we do believe that the complex structure of classical music may be good for your baby's brain while it's forming pathways and connecting synapses. "Twinkle, Twinkle Little Star" and "Hush Little Baby" are enchanting delights that baby will enjoy, especially if Mommy or Daddy sings along.

When my son was a baby, I found a rendition of The Beatles for babies enjoyable. They make lullaby renditions of rock bands, such as Aerosmith, Queen, Green Day, and even AC/DC. Check out *www.rockabyebabymusic.com* to hear a sample before purchasing. For country-music fans, *www.hushabyebabymusic.com* has lullaby renditions of Johnny Cash, Garth Brooks, Dolly Parton, and even newcomer Carrie Underwood. You may find some tunes to make both you and your baby smile.

How Loud Should Baby's Music Be?

Well, not so low that the baby is straining to hear it, and not too loud, to a point where she isn't enjoying it. Also, don't leave music on 24/7, thinking this will constantly stimulate the baby's brain and make her brilliant. If you play music constantly, your baby will start to block it out and get the idea that music is not important or special. If your baby looks stressed because of music, make sure the tempo isn't too fast or escalating at too dramatic a speed. Some classical music is too emotional and complex for their little ears.

In the Car

While I'm the first to admit I love to blare music while I drive, it's not appropriate to blast your baby's sensitive ears. Also, it's okay to be "hip" and "down" with the latest music, but your baby does not need to be exposed to adult content, such as Marilyn Manson, Eminem, or Britney's latest and greatest. A lot of parents want to be cool and "fit the baby into their world," not vice versa. However, consider the impression on your baby's brain when picking his musical introduction to the world. Music he doesn't understand can be scary or alarming, creating a stressful environment. You're conditioning your baby for a successful life of musical enjoyment, so stick with the baby tunes and rock out on your baby-free time.

Tactile Considerations

Baby's bedding should be soft and smooth. Babies that are sensitive to touch will be uncomfortable on coarse fabric that has ridges or bumps. Using "The Princess and the Pea" theory, a stuffed animal or blanket could disturb your little angel's rest. In the story, the princess can't sleep because there is a pea underneath one of her mattresses. While extreme, you get the idea. Something tiny, bumpy, or rough that rubs up against your baby's delicate skin may irritate your baby. Think more about your baby's comfort when choosing bedding, rather than cute decorations. It's okay to be less fashionable and more functional. Choose bedding that is extra-soft, and put her in soft, comfortable pajamas or sleep sacks. Make sure you do not cover your baby with a blanket until she is able to move herself around in the crib or roll over. That way, if she pulls the blanket over her head, she is able to pull it off by herself. Again, there should be no toys or stuffed animals in the bed with her, especially once she starts rolling over and moving in her sleep.

Long Live the Rocking Chair

Many sleep experts will tell you NOT to rock your child, as he will become dependent on the motion to fall asleep. What these experts fail to mention is that rocking with your child in the rocking chair has many wonderful benefits. Ashley Monagu, author of *Touching: The Human Significance of the Skin,* states that rocking is believed to increase cardiac output (the amount of blood pumped through the heart per minute) and aid in circulation, respiration, and digestion, among other things. You can help your baby relieve gas by moving the fluids in baby's intestine back and forward while rocking, aiding in the breakdown and absorption of nutrients. Almost every area of skin is stimulated while you're holding your baby and rocking, and you're moving the inner-ear fluids for vestibular input, as well. So rock on!

Make sure to pick a rocking chair with nontoxic wood (see the next section for more detail) and one that is ergonomically correct, as your back will ache if the chair isn't comfortable to sit in for extended periods of time. You should consider purchasing a rocking footrest to accompany the rocking chair or a stool to rest your feet on in front of the rocking chair for additional support.

Nontoxic Nursery Furniture

When purchasing or borrowing furniture for your baby's nursery, examine the quality of the items, as well as any glue used in its assembly. Does it have a chemical smell? Perhaps it is emitting toxic gaseous fumes. Is it fake wood? Is there glue keeping it together, instead of nails or screws? While formaldehyde is a natural compound in all wood, it's toxic when used as an adhesive in carpets and plywood. Perhaps you could opt for bare wood that has not been treated with sealants. Avoid plastic furniture that contains PVC (polyvinyl chloride), which has been linked to numerous adverse health effects. PVC pipes are used for plumbing because the product is cheap and can easily withstand temperatures and waste, but we suggest you keep it out of baby's bedroom! This compound is being phased out of household items and baby toys and has been removed from the interior of cars. Manufacturers now perceive PVC products to be a serious health risk, so look out for your baby, too. Just because it can be found at your local store *does not mean* it's safe.

Bedding

Mattresses made of natural materials, such as cotton or wool, are supposed to carry the least amount of toxins and chemicals. There are organic baby mattresses available that are made with no formaldehyde or polyurethane. Isn't it strange that we have to pay extra to avoid having these poisons in our bedding?! One day, as society becomes more eco-friendly and "green," organic, nontoxic bedding will hopefully be the only option.

If you have severe allergies and suspect your baby might have them too, one way to keep allergens and dust mites at bay is through allergy-free bedding. There are protective covers available to place over your baby's mattress. There are organic cotton sheets and linens for babies. Try to avoid anything that has been treated chemically, such as fabric that is "permanent press" or "waterproof." If you plan on sleeping together in the same bed, maybe now is the time to invest in a mattress cover for your family bed. The more you can do to protect your baby from toxins, the better. Why? Because toxins may affect your baby's brain development, immune system, and sensory systems. The toxins can be absorbed through your baby's skin while lying on a sheet, on a mattress, and in a crib, and she can inhale toxins through the air she breathes.

Must-Haves

After conferring with other moms, I've put together a "Must-Have Baby Kit" in the Appendix to help you prepare the essential items you'll need when you bring your baby home from the hospital. There's a lot to remember with a newborn, so hopefully this Kit will make things just a little bit easier for you!

Organizing Your Home

You need to think not only about the baby's nursery, but about the rest of your home, as well. Both inside and outside your home, your yard and patio included, are going to be your baby's sanctuary. This will be where she learns, plays, and grows. We encourage you to make your home as sensory friendly as possible for both you and your baby.

Your Bedroom

Where will the baby be sleeping when you first bring him home? Many parents choose to have a bassinet by their bed or even have the baby sleep in the bed with them. This can be easy and convenient when your newborn wakes every few hours to feed. Moms can even breast-feed in a side-lying position, and then it's back to sleep for everyone! Think about if you have to get up in the middle of the night to get to your baby. You don't want to trip on your husband's work boots left in the doorway, because trust me—you will be TIRED!

Living Room

Think about your living room. This may be where you spend a lot of time with your new baby during the day. Are the lights really bright? Can they be dimmed, or can you turn floor lamps on instead of over-head lights? You want to help provide a calm environment for your baby, especially when he is feeding or when you lay him on his back on the floor. Those bright overhead lights can be overwhelming. This is not to say that you always have to have your house dark by any means. When your child is first born, the lights will not bother him too much, and you can have some lights on even in the nursery. As he grows and his eyes develop, however, he can become more sensitive to light, or his eyes may adjust nicely and he may not show any distress to bright lights overhead.

How is the natural lighting in your home? Does the living room receive a lot of sunlight in the morning? This might be a great place to have a tummy-time area for your newborn to help get on a daytime-waking and nighttime-sleeping schedule.

What about those super-strong plug-in air fresheners or fragrant candles that usually smell so nice to us as adults? Those may be too much for your newborn, and you should take into consideration what scents you have in the rooms where the baby will be spending time. Sometimes sensory sensitivities to smells can affect things like nursing. Try nontoxic alternatives, like dropping a little bit of an essential oil on cotton balls and placing them in your heating and air-conditioning vents. Your entire home will smell fresh, without irritating your baby's nose.

Nursing/Feeding Station

You will most likely feed your baby in the living room during the day, unless you feel more comfortable in the nursery. Set up an area where you may comfortably feed your baby with a pillow for support, and a place to keep a glass of water nearby for you, as nursing can be dehydrating. Having a feeding station downstairs if your baby's nursery is upstairs is helpful too, if you're downstairs and your baby needs to eat immediately.

MOM TIP: If you enjoy having your baby take a nap on your chest after feeding, or maybe Daddy likes to enjoy this snuggle time, you can use one of those C-shaped travel pillows to keep your neck from getting stiff. A lot of times, the baby is so cozy that you don't want to move and risk waking the baby or ruining this special time, so having the travel pillow close by can come in very handy and save your neck.

Changing Station

While you will most likely have a complete diaper-changing station in your baby's nursery, it will serve you to have a smaller station set up either downstairs or in your living room. All you need is a basket with diapers, creams, wipes, or whatever items you choose to use, but having access to these items without having to climb the stairs or leave the room can make your life easier at times.

Bathrooms

If you need to get your plumbing fixed, do so before the baby arrives. Drano is a potent concoction that is great for unclogging your drain but is not good for your baby's sensory systems. Take care of any construction that may need to be done to make your bathroom sanitary and functioning for you and your household. Is your sewage backed up? Does rust spew out of your pipes when you turn on the sink? Do you have cleaning products scattered about? Is there mold?

Where are your toiletries put away? Where do you keep your razors? Is your tile slippery in the bathtub or on the bathroom floor? Do you plug your hairdryer in above the bathroom sink and let it drape over the toilet? Rethink how you're going to maneuver in your bathroom while you're tending to a newborn.

Kitchen

Again, make sure your plumbing is in proper working condition. Kitchens are often the hub of the household, and you and your baby may be spending a lot of your time there. Put away the sharp objects and hazardous equipment and prepare for a kid-friendly atmosphere.

Where is your baby's high chair? Does she have a view of your cooking area? Is it set up in a location where the dogs can run through and knock her over?

Clutter

Clear away any clutter from the frequented areas of your home and make sure you have a pathway to the bathroom, kitchen, and, most importantly, wherever the baby is sleeping. Better yet, clear out your entire home while you're nesting. Clutter not only takes up space in your home, it also takes up space in your mind. Have you ever noticed that people with a lot of clutter are usually the same people who lose their keys, are always late, and often don't think clearly? Throw out, donate, and give away items that you don't need or no longer want. Make room for your new life with your baby and for the items that will come as your family grows and grows up.

If you have so much clutter that you don't know where to start, ask a professional for help. There are people who organize for a living, and they will not only clear out your home, they will provide you with tools to help keep the clutter at bay. There are also books, Web sites, and television shows on how to declutter your home. If you don't need it, get rid of it. Why? Because too much "stuff" is hard on your senses, as well as on your baby's sensory system. It's amazing how many items we have that were impulse purchases and are outdated and no longer used. Do you have a computer from 1994 that won't start up? Recycle it—you may even make some money! If you're emotionally connected to the items, perhaps you can talk to a psychologist about why you need the possessions and learn how to let them go.

Baby-Proofing

It's always best to be safe rather than sorry. Safety is paramount when you have a baby. We recommend that you start baby-proofing your home before your baby arrives. Plug in the outlet covers, install the safety locks on the doors, and get your pool gate up. Even though your baby will not come out walking and getting into things, it will happen before you know it, and you will have less time to baby-proof once your baby is on the go. The evolutionary process of being a parent is that you will think of new ways to protect your baby as you get used to being a parent. All of a sudden, earthquake-proofing your flat-screen TV so that it can't fall on an unsuspecting baby will make sense to you.

There are hundreds of baby-proofing products on the market. While some of these are useful, others can be more of a pain than a help. Start by locking away your cleaning products and sharp kitchen utensils and placing gates in the stairways. Start living as if your baby has arrived and be a safety detective. Lie down on the ground and look at things from a baby's perspective. What could you get into? Could that plant fall off that speaker if you bumped into it while learning to crawl? The most important part of safety is prevention. Think ahead.

A lot of baby- and child-proofing is simply clearing paths and putting items away. Notice I didn't say out of reach! Babies start climbing at around a year old, and a tempting object will encourage them to use their toy box as a scaffold as they climb your entertainment center. If the items are valuable to you, put them in a safe place, boxed in the attic or garage, or in storage. Maybe you can keep these items at your parents' house or a friend's home if you don't have space.

Baby-proofing your home will put you at ease. As you will find, it is a challenge to take a baby to family member's house that isn't baby-proofed. You'll spend all your time there keeping your child's hands from yanking on the tablecloth, as the table is loaded with breakable plates. By creating a safe environment for your baby to grow up in, you are giving yourself a sense of peace.

We're big on safety, following manufacturers' manuals, and doing research to make the best choices for your family. While some restrictions or rules may seem extreme, remember that many of those disclaimers are written because children have been hurt in the past. Yes, *someone* must have used the hairdryer in the bathtub!

Play Station

You may want a designated place for your baby to play, both on his back and on his tummy. Pick an area with natural light, if possible, and choose a location where you can get down on the floor and have eye contact with your baby. If you enjoy watching your soap operas in the afternoon, make a place for your baby close to your chair or couch and start a daily ritual of playtime.

Most babies accumulate mountains of toys from your family, friends, and coworkers. Unlike the toys you purchase, these will be the trucks with loud sirens, the annoying water flutes, and the toy with chipping paint from China that your baby wants to chew on. People who do not have children usually give the worst baby gifts; however, they're well meaning, and it is a kind gesture. Stack those toys in the garage or donate them to Goodwill after sending out your thank-you cards. Keep the baby's play space limited to the toys that encourage sensory stimulation and are good for your baby's development. Your baby does not need many toys to keep him entertained. Pick a few to keep in your play station and rotate them out as needed.

Vaccines

Just saying the word "vaccines" can start a heated debate amongst parents. There are the definite "anti-vaccine" crowds, the "pro-vaccine" armies, and the "greener, safer vaccine" camps. We suggest that, just like anything else in parenting, you educate yourself and know the pros, the cons, the risks, and the benefits before your baby is born, as your baby will most likely receive his first Hepatitis B vaccination at birth.

Learn about the contents of the vaccines, just as you would learn about what your baby's food is made of. Many vaccinations are made from eggs (chicken embryos), so knowing if your baby has a food allergy may be important.

Find out about different vaccination schedules and why there are options. Don't make your decision based on fear—fear via either ad campaigns or social pressure. According to the online newsroom for the Centers for Disease Control at *cdc.gove/media/pressre/2010/r100429.com,* only about 40% of Americans received flu vaccinations this year, which was up from 33% in previous years. With that low of a percentage getting vaccinated, the "herd mentality" doesn't really apply as much as some would like you to think. Polio and the measles are not rampant in our country, with less than 50% of the population getting vaccinated.

What vaccinations do other countries use? What are their infant mortality rates? What are your school district's policies for allowing children to enroll without vaccinations? What about your daycare? How have the babies in your family reacted to shots recently? Have your nieces and nephews had no reaction? Or do they get sick and develop hives? Research. Ask. It's your responsibility.

A few things that we do know for sure: Do not give your baby Tylenol before or after being vaccinated. The Tylenol reacts within your child's system to spread the vaccine further through the bloodstream, which is not a good thing. So if your child has a fever after being vaccinated, please don't give him Tylenol—ask your doctor for other suggestions. Also, do not vaccinate your baby if she's already sick and has a weakened immune system. Please note that there are no scientific studies regarding the health of your baby if she's given several shots at one time, so if your argument is science, please collect scientific facts for both sides of the debate. There are many with contradicting outcomes, depending on who is paying for the study and research. You may have to make several trips to your doctor to get one shot each time, but weigh out the options between safety and convenience.

As an occupational therapist who sees many types of families coming into my office that have been affected in some way from vaccines, I try to suggest that parents spread them out and don't get more than two shots in one day. Remember that the MMR vaccine is three vaccinations given in one shot. Many doctors and nurses will tell you they have to give your baby nine shots at once because you are behind schedule, but remember that this is not the law, and YOU can decide what you want for your child. Also remember that vaccines are a drug that you are injecting into a small baby or child, so make sure you have educated yourself before you make any decisions.

Books about vaccinations that we recommend are: *Vaccine Safety Manual: For Concerned Families and Health Practitioners,* by Neil Miller, and *The Vaccine Book: Making the Right Decision for Your Child,* by Robert W. Sears, MD, FAAP. Web sites we recommend are *www.cdc.gov* and *www.thinktwice.com.*

If you can, try to think, plan, and educate yourself without being reactionary (if that is even possible as a new parent). Good luck!

CHAPTER TWO

Your Newborn
(0 to 6 Months)

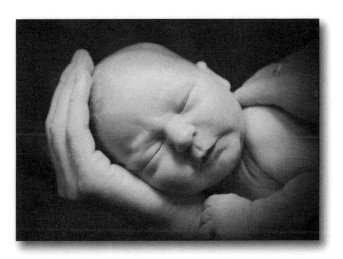

There is nothing as beautiful as a parent and their newborn.
BRITT'S NEPHEW, JACKSON, IN DADDY'S HANDS

Bonding with Your Baby

FINALLY, YOUR BABY HAS ARRIVED! CONGRATULATIONS—YOU MADE IT. NOW the fun begins! Don't feel bad if you don't remember everything exactly as you've read or been told—your baby is resilient, and so are you. Just give your baby love and attention and meet her daily needs, and you will both figure out the rest along the way. We hope to provide you with tips and tools to use as you and your baby learn about each other.

Baby's Sight

You and your baby will first connect through eye-love.[1] Parents are known to gaze into their infant's eyes for long periods of time, which naturally forms a deep connection. Since babies can't do much other than look at their parents, this is an instinctual way for the two of you to bond. Your baby is processing his external world, which primarily consists of you. Building a sense of security and attachment is something that will stay with your baby for his entire lifetime.

Soon, your baby will match your expressions—smiling if you smile, frowning if you frown, and eventually sticking his tongue out if you do. This is known as *mirroring* and is another way to make a connection with your baby.

Peek-a-boo is a good game to play with babies to connect with them and to teach presence and absence. Your baby is truly surprised with your appearance and disappearance. The surprise turns into anticipation when your baby makes the connection that you're going to return. This game can be helpful in building a solid foundation for a lifetime of connecting and reconnecting with your child.

NOTE: *If your child has a medical condition with his eyes, it does not mean you're not going to build a connection with your child. Nature and your baby's other senses will ensure that proper bonding occurs!*

Baby's Hearing

Parents instinctually raise their voice pitch an octave or two when talking to their baby. Why? Because newborns seem to prefer high-pitched tones and will turn their heads and give attention to the sound. Something about a parent's soothing, loving voice creates a desire to listen to it and to be open and receptive. Babies tend to turn away from a voice that carries anger, depression, or anxiety.

Your baby's life begins in the womb, where she has had the constant comfort of Mom's heartbeat and voice. She is then welcomed into the outside world, where her auditory system must adapt and clear itself of prenatal fluids. The adjustment takes about 4 months, while she acclimates to the airborne mode of auditory perception. To aid with this transition, mothers (parents and caregivers) are encouraged to sing to the baby while holding her, which stimulates many areas of her brain and her ears simultaneously. This is known as body-to-body transmission of sound through vibration of the bone structure, which is similar to the prenatal way a baby receives sound from her mother.[2] Don't worry if you don't have a great singing voice—your baby won't mind!

Your baby is also listening and teaching himself to talk. This process stems from the baby realizing that his laugh and cry is his and can be manipulated. He learns that he can imitate sounds around him and then make the astonishing connection that the sound "Ma-ma" will bring his mommy closer to him.

It is unfortunate that ear infections are so common in children during this crucial stage of auditory development. A baby's ears and his vestibular system are not only absorbing language, but the ears are also receptors of movements, which have an energizing effect on the baby's rapidly developing brain. The ears can also contribute to the future development of motor functions. Besides being painful, ear infections affect a baby's mood, making him clingy and agitated. Wouldn't you be that way if you were suffering? I'd cling to my mommy too!

Baby's Vestibular System

Beyond the five senses that are commonly known (sight, sound, taste, touch, and smell), the vestibular system is another sense that we will explore throughout this book. When we talk about the vestibular sense, we're talking about the very complex system that regulates our balance and movement, which also affects our vision and posture (being able to stand upright). The vestibular system is governed by the fluid of the inner ear, which lets us know if we are right-side up or upside-down. Like all the other amazing functions of our bodies that work without our attention, the vestibular system adapts and changes according to our environment. Our job as parents and caregivers is to guide the development of a child's vestibular system and to watch for signals that the system needs adapting or repair.

Baby's Touch and Proprioception

Our skin is our largest organ, and it performs many functions. It protects our internal world from the external world, feeds us information about the environment and our temperature, and allows us to feel pressure and vibrations as sensations to help us regulate where we are in space. The skin offers many more amazing contributions, but these are the duties we're focusing on to explain how skin affects your baby. The skin allows your baby to feel and touch, enabling skin-to-skin contact and bonding with Mom and Dad. This contact can calm your baby, and holding your baby on your chest to feel and hear your heartbeat will teach your baby to self-calm.

Think about the millions of receptors on your baby's skin. By holding him, this gives each of those receptors feedback and pressure, which lets your baby know where he ends and where you begin. This feedback is referred to as proprioception, and it is an internal sense that allows the body to know where each body part is in reference to another. For example, this system lets you know where your hand is in relation to your foot and allows you to walk without having to look down at your feet. If a baby's proprioceptive system is off, she will feel as though her limbs are dangling in space, without any connection. Another example of poor proprioception is falling off a curb because you misjudged how close you were to it.

This is one reason babies like to be swaddled. The pressure from the blankets is like the womb, giving the baby feedback about where his body is.

It has been proven time and time again that babies crave contact with their parents and/or caregivers. They need this to be able to build trust in their parents and trust in the world. This contact is a crucial component in building a solid lifelong foundation for your child. Without trust, your child will never feel that he is good enough, that the world is there for him, and that his needs will be met. If your baby is crying to be held, he may need that pressure, security, and feedback for his body. He doesn't understand that he's feeling alone and flailing in space—he just knows instinctually that he needs to be held. We're not saying you have to hold your baby all the time—that's extreme. However, holding your baby and having skin-to-skin contact is vital.

You cannot spoil a baby by holding him—we are strict believers in this rule. You can also not spoil a baby by meeting his needs—feeding, changing, and providing for him. How would you feel if you couldn't feed yourself, soothe yourself, burp yourself, or change yourself, and your caregiver didn't help you? What message do you want to send your baby?

If your baby has an aversion to being held and prefers to be left alone, perhaps you should experiment with different types of touch to see if there is a more peaceful touch your baby prefers. Sometimes, deep pressure is more comforting for baby, while a soft touch can be painful. You have to work with your baby to find out how his skin reacts and what messages are being sent to his brain. We'll go deeper into this subject later on.

Baby's Taste

Babies explore the outside world with their mouths. For the first few years of development, babies are known to place all sorts of objects into their mouths. Why? Because they are receiving input and information about textures, tastes, and the way things generally feel in their mouths. If a toy is dirty or falls on the floor in a public place, just wash it off. Mouthing objects is a normal part of development.

Sucking is a natural reflex that we are born with to help us survive. Some babies take a little time to learn how to latch on and get a hang of the suck-swallow-breathe pattern. Once they get this down, feeding becomes much easier. Babies also have a nonnutritive suck for their fingers, hands, or pacifiers. Sucking is rhythmical and soothing, which usually helps calm babies down and even helps them fall asleep.

Many babies take to a pacifier, or "binky," and some babies prefer their fingers or nothing at all. Sometimes, even in the womb, you can see a baby sucking on her thumb. Binkies are soothing and are a good way to help your baby calm down. They can also help strengthen your baby's oral-motor skills down the road. Binkies are relatively easy to get rid of when the child gets older, as opposed to sucking her thumb— sometimes you won't be able to avoid it if the child really wants to suck her fingers or thumb.

Babies that are born orally defensive will most likely reject plastic pacifiers and prefer the breast. These babies want to nurse constantly and don't wean easily. Don't worry, there are simple things you can do that will help both you and your baby! We'll give you all sorts of skills to work on with your baby in our "picky eaters" chapter.

Baby's Sense of Smell

Don't forget that perfect little nose! While smell is a sense that doesn't get a lot of attention in comparison to sight and hearing, it should be noted that the human olfactory sense is quite powerful. Without knowing it, smell helps us decide another person's likability and emotional state. On a subconscious level, babies can smell if a person is a stranger or a friend.

Many children have a strong sense of smell and are highly sensitive to certain smells. When bringing home an infant, examine carefully what types of smells you have in your house.

Do you have a lot of strong-smelling candles? Plug-in air fresheners in the outlets? Pets with litter boxes, or dander, or muddy paw prints? Do you have mold in your home, either because it is an older home or because you live in a damp area? This could cause allergies. Did you recently paint the baby's room? Do you burn incense in your home?

Take all of these things into consideration when you bring your newborn home for the first time, with her sensitive little nose and olfactory system. We suggest that you use all-natural cleaning products, and don't use any cleaning chemicals while your baby is nearby. Kirman Kleen is a great brand that is nontoxic and offers unscented products, from personal items like shampoo and lotion to cleaning supplies. Target carries Seventh Generation nontoxic cleaning products. Read labels, and find out what is in your household products. "Green" is in for a reason! It's easier and more affordable than ever to clean without harming your baby. We also suggest that you wait until she is asleep in her own room before you mop the kitchen floor or polish the coffee table. Use all-natural products to deodorize or make your home smell nice—for instance, natural, lightly scented candles. However, never leave candles burning where your baby could reach them!

Parents, if you smoke—you stink! Smoke stays in your hair, on your clothes, and on your skin. Gum-chewing, musky perfume, and smoke-removal sprays only add to the nasal poison. If you must smoke, NEVER SMOKE AROUND YOUR BABY, and please—shower often and wash your hair. Otherwise, your baby will inhale the toxins when you pick her up and hold her face next to your neck. Talk to your doctor about ways to stop smoking, including nicotine gum and patches, hypnotherapy, and any other viable alternatives.

Bathing, Changing Diapers, Dressing, and Swaddling

Bath Time

When preparing to bathe your baby for the first time, think about the water temperature, the room temperature, the texture of the washcloth you are using, and the types of soap you are using. There are many choices available, but we recommend using something natural with no chemicals and no scent. You can use your elbow to test the temperature of the water to make sure it is not too hot. There is also a rubber-duck toy that can tell you whether the water temperature is just right for your baby. If you use one, always double-check the water temperature yourself, just to be safe. Be sure the room is nice and warm so that when you take the baby out of the sink or tub, he is not moving into an extremely different temperature. Wrap him up in a soft towel and hold him close for comfort.

When you first bring your baby home, you can sponge-bathe him until his umbilical cord has fallen off, and until a circumcision has healed, if your baby had one. You will only need to bathe your baby a few times a week—you don't want to dry out his delicate skin. If you bathe your child a few times a week or even sponge-bathe him, you can use soap if there is dirt or food on him or if you are cleaning his private areas, hands, and face. However, you can also just use water. When washing around the eyes of a newborn, use a sterile cotton ball that you have dipped in warm water, and gently wash around the eye area.

Always remember, it doesn't matter whether you are bathing your baby in a sink or bath chair or in a regular tub—NEVER leave him alone, even for a minute. Gather all of your materials before beginning bath time.

When bathing a baby in water, be cautious of how far you tip her head back, so you do not strain her neck when you are gently pouring water over her head. Make sure you are not bending over too far and straining your back. You are going to be carrying around this little baby and all of her accoutrements for a while, and you want your body to be strong and pain-free. If you are bathing her in the kitchen sink, think about sitting on a tall stool to save some of your energy, since you are going to be busy for the next few months!

Changing Diapers

As all parents know, changing diapers can be effortless at times, and extremely complicated at others, depending on where you are and how your baby is feeling. To make this common practice as painless as possible, pay attention to your baby's cues. Is your baby cold as you take off her pajamas? Is she covered in fecal matter and urine? Does she have a diaper rash? Does she want to be naked? It's often a matter of trial and error, and just when you think you've got it down, your baby will change and grow into wanting something else.

Use a calming voice when laying the child down to change her. If she acts like she is scared to lie back, then slowly lower her to the changing table or floor, while holding her head and giving her as much physical support as you can. Think about how far you are lowering her. If you are standing up and you are going to lay her on the floor, think about how far that is from your baby's perspective! IT'S A LONG WAY DOWN! If you are just going from standing to the changing table, it may not be as bad. Or, if you are standing, kneel down, then sit, then lay her down on the floor to change her. This helps your baby to gradually adjust to the gravitational changes that you just made and gives her more time to allow her body and mind to adjust.

Some babies like to be naked and squirm around on the changing table, but some babies don't want to be undressed completely. You can just quickly take off his bottoms and unsnap his Onesie if he has one on, and then change him. However, often a baby has what we call a "blaster," and he is covered from head to toe in poop. What can you do except strip the baby down and clean him up completely before putting a new diaper on? For your sake and your baby's, do it as calmly and as quickly as possible. You can even sing to your baby while you clean him up. Don't make him feel dirty for needing to be changed— enjoy these natural and sometimes funny situations, and use the time to bond with your baby, even if he is screaming and fussy. You will get through it!

Some mothers like to use a "wipe warmer," so the wipes are not cold on the baby's bottom. If you choose not to use disposable wipes, soft washcloths and warm water work just as well, and you may avoid irritation to your baby's sensitive skin. A cream for diaper rash can also be helpful—try an all-natural one, like Burt's Bees, or some mothers like Boudreaux's Butt Paste (yes, that's its real name!). Make sure you wipe your baby from the front toward the back to avoid getting any poop in any unwanted places, and clean thoroughly. Wiping from front to back helps avoid bladder infections in little girls.

Now for that age-old decision—cloth diapers or disposables? First of all, we'd like to advise you to please take your baby's sensory systems into consideration. Some babies prefer the feel of cloth diapers, while others prefer the drier feel of disposable diaper absorption. Remember that cloth diapers are sometimes covered with a plastic casing to go over the diaper. Some babies prefer the looser feel of cloth, while others prefer the tight, snug feel of the disposable. We personally do not have a preference, especially now that we've learned that disposable diapers can be melted down and recycled out of landfills with modern technology. This is exciting news for us and for future generations, thanks to companies such as Knowaste and CleanTech Biofuels, amongst other eco-friendly superheroes. Please note that the biodegradable diapers have absorbent gels that may be just as toxic as disposable diapers.

Getting Dressed

When you are dressing your baby, consider the weather and temperature outside, and dress him in layers so that if it's warm inside and cold outside, you can add or take away layers as needed. Babies have a more sensitive body temperature than we do as adults. Look to see if your baby is hot or sweating, or feel his hands and feet to see if they are cold and need socks. Also, when dressing your baby, think soft and snuggly, with no tags poking at him and nothing too tight and restrictive, especially when he hits the 4-month-old mark and is starting to move around more, roll, and sit.

When your child begins to crawl, make sure he has comfortable pants that give him enough room, and if you are concerned about carpet burns on his knees or feet, dress him in soft pants and socks. Some children will begin to "bear walk," with their hands on the ground, their bottoms in the air, and their feet following behind them. It is easier to do this without socks on so they don't slip.

Bring along extra clothing for your baby, in case of diaper leaks and other messy situations. Babies tend to need fresh clothing throughout the day. It is okay for your baby to be naked sometimes, too—maybe to air out a diaper rash or to feel the warm sun on her body for a moment. Don't forget the sunscreen! Your baby may also "go potty" while naked, so be ready for clean-up or keep your baby in a diaper!

If you live in a warmer climate, your baby may want to be naked (or in diaper) while she is at home or while playing. It's not necessarily a sign that your baby has tactile sensitivities if she prefers to let it all hang loose. If your baby has an aversion, you'll know by the way she arches her back when you try to dress her, and also if she thrashes about in a maniacal way. For these babies, dress them quickly if possible

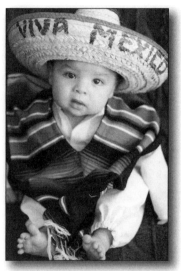

Viva la Mexico!
ALEXANDER'S FIRST
CELEBRATION

(while still being safe) and only put them in soft, breathable fabrics with limited seams, zippers, and anything else that may bother their skin.

In colder climates, put the lighter, softer clothes closest to the baby's skin before bundling her up in layers for winter. Watch for seams in your baby's socks and mittens that could rub on her sensitive limbs. You might go with more sack-style attire if your baby is difficult to dress.

Dressing Up Baby

Oh what fun it can be to dress up your baby for an event! Whether it's a frilly dress with ruffles, a miniature tuxedo for your sister's wedding, or perhaps a special outfit for a religious ceremony, dressing your baby up in cute clothes always makes for an adorable photo opportunity. Halloween costumes are often hard to resist, as every baby looks precious as a bumblebee, or, in my son's case, "Piglet." What we need to remember is that these outfits are not usually very baby friendly. They're bulky, they can be hot, and some have a zillion seams rubbing up against and irritating your baby's sensitive skin. If you must dress your baby in one of these outfits, try to keep the time they're forced to wear it to a mini-mum. Don't put a heavy hat or hoodie on your baby if it's straining his neck (that lion's mane might not be a good idea). Try to find a costume that allows your baby's skin to breathe and think about putting your baby in a soft Onesie under the less-gentle fabrics. Be sure to take lots of photos, as your baby will grow out of this ensemble quickly!

Swaddling

Chances are, upon your baby's birth, the hospital nurse will swaddle your baby in a triangular piece of fabric, tucking the baby's arms and legs into a snug wrap, leaving his head out and safely away from the blanket. Swaddling your child can be comforting, and many babies like to be swaddled from day one. They will start to let you know if they do not enjoy this feeling or if they crave it. Some babies will slowly begin to wiggle their arms out, one at a time, and then kick the swad-dled blanket off their legs, but other children sleep well in that tight little cocoon. Listen to what your baby is telling you to know how much he likes being swaddled.

My son had to be swaddled as often as possible, or he'd flail and scream. He wanted to be held tightly, and in order to get him to sleep, he had to be securely wrapped up in his cocoon. I later learned that this was related to his vestibular system being "off," which gave him gravitational insecurities. He constantly felt like he was falling. What a scary feeling, especially for a baby!

There are items on the market to help with baby swaddling, such as the "Swaddlekeeper" at *www.swaddlekeeper.com*. This is a blanket with built-in support for baby's neck, and the sides of the blanket have Vel-cro to keep the baby wrapped tightly, while her legs are loose. For a super-tight, all-over snug fit, you can try the miracle blanket at *www.miracleblanket.com*. Remember, there are always good, old-fash-ioned baby blankets that work great, too!

Some babies will grow out of swaddling around 4-5 months of age, and they can learn how to self-soothe and fall back asleep when they awaken in the night. Other babies have a hard time self-soothing and rely on the tightly swaddled blanket around them.

One mom told me how her son was swaddled until 8 months of age, and she had extreme difficulty getting him to soothe himself back to sleep when he would wake up in the night. She is planning on doing things differently with her second baby. She's encouraging her to learn how to self-soothe and calm, so that she will not be doing battle with an 8-month-old screaming baby, trying to teach her (the hard way) how to comfort herself. However, The Baby Whisperer, Tracy Hogg, recommends that parents swaddle for as long as a baby craves it. All moms go through trial and error and end up working it all out one way or another.

Baby in Motion

Babies used to be carried by their mothers constantly. Whether Mom was working in a field or gathering food, the baby was strapped to her. Naturally, having the baby close to his mother in that way helped him learn to regulate his body and internal systems in a rhythmical pattern, similar to his mother's. Today, babies are often transported in synthetic carriers, strollers, car seats, and swings, so they do not get the same natural programming to their sensory systems. Here are some examples of modern motions that babies are subjected to and ways to help their sensory systems process and adapt to external information.

Please note: We're not dismissing strollers, swings, and the like. We love our gadgets like everyone else, and I, personally, can't live without my cup holders and extra storage space for my purse! As we talk about sensory needs, just know that we're not asking you to give up any of your devices completely.

I know it can be convenient to take the whole baby seat out of the car, carry it into the grocery store, and place it in the shopping cart to do your grocery shopping. However, consider this experience from the perspective of your child. Now all she has to look at is the tops of the shelves and the lights in her eyes. She hears voices but cannot see where they come from. While it can be more difficult to strap your child into an upright carrier that you can wear around the store (either on your front or your back), give it a try sometimes! Then your baby can see the world as we do, in an upright position where she can learn about the sights, sounds, smells, and social interactions going on around her.

Motion, the Vestibular System, and Gravitational Insecurity

The sense of falling or feeling like your feet are further from the ground than they are is called *gravitational insecurity.* If your baby becomes physically sick when he is moved too fast or moved in a certain way, which his body cannot process correctly, this may be a sign that his vestibular system is not functioning properly. I know a child who always got sick when he rode in a car. Every time his parents tried to take him anywhere, he arched his head back and screeched, as if he was being tortured. He often vomited when the car was in motion. He also cried and clung to his parents if they tried to lay him down in the crib, sit him in a swing, or initiate any other type of movement. After years of occupational therapy, which we will discuss in the following chapters, he still cannot tolerate a ride at Disneyland or being on a boat. He does, however, enjoy car rides and can now ride on a train. It's all about baby steps!

Balls

Some babies seem to calm down when you gently bounce them while sitting on an exercise ball. Find the right size for you, and make sure it is fully blown up. You want your hips and knees to be at a 90° angle when sitting on the ball while you bounce your baby. You can hold her against your shoulder to give her head support. The bouncing moves the fluid in her inner ears, which is good for her vestibular system.

My son particularly liked being held in the cradle hold (his head in the crook of my arm, with my other arm wrapped around him) while I bounced with him on a ball. The gentle bouncing soothed him to sleep. An added benefit of bouncing is that it's good for Mommy's legs and tummy!

If you're looking for ways for Daddy or your parenting partner to help out and bond with the baby, ask him to take shifts bouncing. It can be fun for the baby and gives Daddy time to bond. He can even watch the basketball game if he promises to keep a strong hold and not get distracted.

Body Carriers

The Baby Björn and other wraps are excellent resources for parents and babies. They allow parents to remain mobile with their hands free, while simultaneously comforting their child and exposing him to new environments in a secure position. Babies are able to process new sights, sounds, and sensations while feeling protected by their parent. For parents, they provide support for carrying around the extra weight of a newborn and enable you to be able to continue with your daily duties while keeping your baby close.

Babies who may have gravitational insecurities or difficulty process-ing vestibular input from their environment may want to be wrapped up most of the time and held close to an adult's body. This closeness allows them to learn how to regulate their bodies and process the envi-ronment. If they're extremely sensitive and have a number of sensory issues, this attachment to their parent can help them outgrow some of their sensitivities and also help increase their tolerance to uncomfort-able stimuli, such as crowds, bright lights, or even auditory sensitivities. While we never force a child into an uncomfortable situ-ation, sometimes, if they're close to a parent, babies will slowly adapt to being in a crowd because they want to be with their parent.

Cars, Trucks, Trains, and Planes

Children these days are stimulated constantly. Long ago, children played with sticks, pots, and pans. Now children have DS games (videogames) to play in the car and DVDs to watch while Mom pops into the grocery store. Is this good or bad? We're indifferent. It's part of life, it's progress, it's the way it is—so let's roll with it. That said, please take into account the amount of stimuli your child is being inundated with and adjust accordingly, so that the developing years are positive and fulfilling.

Your baby cannot tell you if she's feeling carsick, so as a parent, you much watch for signs. Is your baby pale and restless? Is she crying and arching her back? Does your child vomit in the car? You should ask your pediatrician to check your child's semicircular canals to see if your baby has an ear infection that may be causing the motion sickness.

Since my child often got carsick, the DVD player was actually a gift. Watching "Baby Einstein" and "Finding Nemo" helped to distract him from his motion sickness. Allowing him to focus on the TV and not on the passing cars, trees, and lights helped his body learn how to regulate itself during the motion of the car ride. You have to do whatever works for your child. For children who are not so sensitive, I encourage parents to only use the TV in the car for long road trips and to talk with their children while driving, or to have them look out the window to see what's going on around them and explore with their eyes. Again, this depends on the child.

When traveling with a baby on public transportation, such as a bus, train, or plane, take into consideration the sounds, smells, sights, and external stimuli that your baby is having to process. Keep your baby close to you if possible and make sure he's dressed comfortably. Don't allow passengers who smell bad or are loud to get in your baby's face or space. Monitor your baby's reactions to movement and make adjustments to comfort your baby, if necessary. If you're flying, understand that the cabin pressure may be hard on your baby's ears. Encourage your baby to suck on a pacifier or have a bottle during take-off and landing to help relieve pressure. Babies don't know to swallow like we do to clear our ears, so if they are drinking or sucking, this will encourage them to swallow.

Do yourself and everyone else on board a favor and keep your baby occupied. Books and travel games are fun ways to keep your baby's attention. Always provide proper snacks and liquids. A happy baby makes for a happier trip for all involved. Many times, parents will tell me that their baby was an angel on the flight out, but coming home was a disaster. Make sure you do not overtire your infant or young child before coming home from a trip. Before you fly, arrange to arrive at the airport early. Make sure your child is well fed and entertained. With any luck, he might even sleep on the plane ride home.

Swings

Swings can be comforting for a young baby. You may have been advised not to let your baby fall asleep in the swing, because you will never get him to sleep in his crib without movement. When you have a child that is difficult to console, however, and he seems to crave that gentle rocking to help him calm down or sleep, there is nothing wrong with rocking him in a rocking chair or putting him in a swing for a little while. The linear (back and forth) movement is calming because it moves the fluid in the inner ear, which activates the vestibular system and soothes the child into a more restful state. Make sure you do not leave your child unattended in a swing, as he can tip over face-first or slip out the bottom of the swing.

There may be a chance that a child does not enjoy this movement. A child that is overresponsive to vestibular input or has gravitational insecurities, for example, would probably not like it.

Feeding Your Baby

Whether you decide to breastfeed or bottle-feed your baby, we support you. It is a personal choice and preference for you and your family. Either way can be a great way to provide nourishment to your baby, and both ways of feeding have their challenges.

Breastfeeding is an excellent source of nutrients and gives the baby the antibodies he needs to have a strong immune system. This is also a great way to bond with your baby. If you bottle-feed, make sure you get the best possible formula for your child. Talk to your pediatrician about what he or she suggests, as there are many brands to choose from.

Your newborn baby will probably want to eat every 2-3 hours, and as she grows bigger, she will eat more at each feeding and feed less often. For early feedings, your baby will probably spend about 5-10 minutes on each breast. If he is taking more than 60 minutes to feed, then he may be having difficulty with sucking and swallowing. If this occurs, you may want to consult a lactation specialist or your pediatrician. When the baby is feeding, you should hear the rhythmical sound of suck, pause, suck, so you know the baby is sucking, swallowing, and breathing.

You will get better results if you feed your baby when he is fully awake. You can talk to him, change his diaper, or play with him to wake him up fully before you feed him.

Take note of where you feed your baby. If you're in a busy room with siblings, noises, and TV, the baby may be distracted and interested in what's going on around him. If you're able, take your baby into a quiet room so he may focus on the task at hand. Sometimes your arms will get tired when you hold your baby while nursing, so use pillows to support the baby and your arms. Make sure you are comfortable, because you will be doing this A LOT!

OCCUPATIONAL THERAPIST TIP: *From a sensory perspective, breastfed babies have more organized sensory systems. They seem to be able to calm themselves more easily, get into a routine more efficiently, and, although they need to wake more often to eat in the beginning, they are able to put themselves back to sleep. However, this does not mean that if you have to bottle-feed, or choose to, that you cannot encourage your baby to have good organizational skills as an infant.*

Breastfeeding

Breastfeeding can be a stressful and frightening experience. You want me to do *what* with my nipple? As a mother who has breastfed, I know it's not always easy, especially at first. I have breast implants and was fearful that I wouldn't be able to breastfeed. A wonderful lactation specialist helped me and my baby get started, and it turned out that I did have a lot of milk available for my baby. The problem was that it was painful. My nipples cracked and bled, and I've since learned that this is quite common. I used lanolin to help with the pain, and, eventually, a few blocked ducts later, my baby and I got into the swing of it. The La Leche League International has tons of great advice, and there are many books devoted to breastfeeding. A favorite of mine was *So That's What They're For! The Definitive Breastfeeding Guide*, written by Janet Tamaro. This book was both humorous and informative and quickly became my daily go-to reference for when yet another breastfeeding issue arose.

MOM AND NEONATAL INTENSIVE-CARE UNIT (NICU) NURSE TIP: *When you are breastfeeding, find a quiet, comfortable place to sit. If your baby's suction is too tight and it is painful, put your little finger (with your nails clipped short) in the side of her mouth to break the suction and get her to latch on again. This is usually a result of improper mouth positioning on your nipple. Consult with a lactation consultant if you are feeling frustrated at any time.*

Most doctors say that breastfeeding should not hurt, and that if it does, seek help. We agree and acknowledge that it really is different for every woman. Some mothers we talked to never felt a tinge of pain, and breastfeeding was a breeze for them—blissful and effortless. For others, it's not as joyous.

Don't give up too easily. Breastfeeding can be very difficult and painful, but many moms report that after 8 to 10 weeks, everything gets so much better. One day, it seems to click into place. The pain subsides, the baby gets the rhythm down, and Mom feels like she is able to bond with her baby and provide her with a good source of nutrients.

What you don't want to do is get so stressed out that the baby senses your anxiety or stress about breastfeeding. You have to do what is best for you, your mental health, and your baby.

Breast Milk from a Bottle

Even if you are breastfeeding, you will more than likely still give your baby a bottle at some point, when someone else needs to feed her. You want to make sure breastfeeding is established before you begin introducing bottles, so give it 3 to 4 weeks. You can pump your breast milk and freeze it, so that you can warm up milk to give your baby later. When choosing a bottle, think about how old your baby is and how much milk she can tolerate at once. You want to choose a slow-flowing nipple to start with that will not overwhelm the baby. Some babies are able to tolerate more milk at one time, and others need a really slow flow of milk so that she does not gag or choke. Talk with your pediatrician and possibly a lactation specialist to decide what is best for your baby.

Breastfeeding in Public

Once you become a pro, breastfeeding in public is a piece of cake. If you're not comfortable at first, feed your baby in the privacy of your vehicle or in a public restroom. There are cover-ups that will help you cover your breast while feeding and allow your baby to breathe while being tucked away. My favorite was the Poochie Nursing Cover, designed by Polka Stripe founder Nikki De La Torre. You can find this at *www.polkastripe.com.* As a mom of four, Nikki knows all about breastfeeding in public, maneuvering those nursing bras with one hand and holding your baby with the other. These nursing covers give you the freedom to hold your baby securely and arrange your bra without giving anyone a peep show. Not that anyone needs to cover up while breastfeeding—it just depends on your comfort level. The more relaxed you are, the easier it is to feed your baby.

Dad/Partner Feeding Time

DAD TIP: *I went with my wife to a breastfeeding class. I didn't think I needed to go at first, but I actually learned more than I expected, and I recommend this class to all my guy friends who are expecting. It gave me a better understanding of what my wife was going through when she was breastfeeding.*

It is important for the father (or partner) to have bonding time with his newborn baby. Sometimes, it seems like only Mom can comfort the baby and bond with him because she is the primary feeder. Dads—it's your turn! You can hold your baby close and feed him a bottle of Mom's breast milk or formula. If you are having difficulty getting him to eat, you can hold a piece of cloth or clothing that has Mom' scent on it while he eats to help him remain calm and want to eat while he's in your arms. You can talk to him gently, but sometimes babies are distracted by noises while they are concentrating on eating. Many babies enjoy a man's deep voice, so go ahead and sing to him—no one is watching or listening, except your little one.

Bottle-Feeding

If you choose to bottle-feed your baby or you are unable to continue breastfeeding for whatever reason, here are some tips on bottle-feeding your child. Again, feeding time is bonding time with your baby, so hold her close in your arms, just as if you were breastfeeding. The question is, "How much do I feed her?" This is a good question, because your breast produces the right amount of milk for the baby. If you are bottle-feeding, you don't know exactly how much formula to make. Remember that your baby's needs will change as she grows, but in general, according to the American Academy of Pediatrics, a baby drinks about 2 ½ ounces of formula or breast milk a day for every pound she weighs. As she grows, she will be able to eat more at one time. Talk to your pediatrician about specific guidelines for your baby.

"How do I know which bottle to use?" Make sure you choose a bottle that is BPA (bisphenol A) free and try various brands to see what your baby likes. For your newborn, have bottles filled with room-temperature water (not cold water!) in your room and have the right amount of formula measured out. That way, when your baby wakes in the night to feed, you can mix the formula and water together and feed your baby immediately.

Start by gently touching the nipple of the bottle to your baby's lips. Allow a drop of milk to come out, so she knows that you are about to feed her. Make sure you tip the bottle up, filling the nipple with milk and keeping air out of the bottle and out of her tummy. If your baby falls asleep while taking a bottle, this signals that she is done for now. If your baby acts fussy while bottle-feeding, stop, and try to burp her before offering the bottle again. She may have gas.

If your baby is gulping down the milk too fast or it's leaking out the side of her mouth, the nipple flow may be too fast for her. Try a slower-flowing nipple. You will find that there are many choices these days in terms of flow. If your baby is struggling to get enough milk and seems to be working too hard to suck, you may want a faster-flowing nipple. Have a few on hand to try until you get the hang of what your baby needs. Again, she will change as she grows, and you can adjust to her needs as you go along.

Another thing you want to do is to have some skin-to-skin contact with your baby, even while bottle-feeding. Hold your baby in your arms as if you were breastfeeding, look into her eyes, and talk to her quietly. This helps form that mother-baby bond that is so special. As you would if you were breastfeeding, switch arms occasionally so that she gets a different visual of you and feels the warmth of your other side. Have your shirt open as you feed her so she gets that valuable skin-to-skin contact.

Swallowing

Here are some common signs of abnormal swallowing during breast-feeding or bottle-feeding. If you notice your baby doing any of these things, consult with your pediatrician.

- Choking
- Coughing
- Making loud gulping sounds
- Discoloring of the face or interruption of breathing
- Regurgitating—bringing the milk back up constantly

Pacifiers (Sucking)

When choosing a pacifier, many families begin with the Soothie or a gumdrop binky, which is smaller and more apt to fit into a newborn's mouth. You can then change to a binky with a different shape at around 6 to 9 months of age, if you choose. Some babies enjoy sucking a pacifier to help soothe and calm them, but some babies will not want it, or they have trouble figuring out how to actually suck on the binky.

OCCUPATIONAL THERAPIST TIP: *One thing you can do to help strengthen your baby's oral-motor skills and suck pattern is to actually dangle the binky just at his lips and tongue and have him work to get it in his mouth fully. If you hold it in his mouth all the time, he may not learn how to suck efficiently enough to keep the binky in his mouth.*

If a baby does not want a binky, he is usually fairly efficient at spitting it out.

The rhythm of your baby's nutritive suck (when he eats) should be about one suck per second. When he is sucking on a binky or his fingers (a nonnutritive suck), the rhythm should be about two sucks per second.

Teething

When a baby is teething, which can begin as early as 3 to 4 months, it can be soothing to suck or chew on a cold teether, which you can pull out of the refrigerator when needed. Your baby may not be able to hold it, so you can hold it for her.

I also recommend using a vibrating toy for teething, which you can start around 4 to 5 months and use all the way through the various teething stages. Babies can hold onto the toy, and when they bite down, the toy gently vibrates and soothes their sore gums.

When you see your baby rubbing his ears, you may think he has an ear infection, but this could also mean he is teething. He can run a fever while teething, and he may not eat as much as he usually does. Teething drops or tablets can help, along with baby Motrin and chilled or vibrating teething toys. Search your local store for teethers and discuss what medicine you can give your baby with your pediatrician.

Sleeping

There is a great deal of pressure put on babies to sleep through the night. As adults, we must remember that a baby does not have to get up in the morning to go to work, and a baby has a tiny stomach and needs nutrients to grow. Your baby's brain and internal systems are working really hard to develop and adapt to this new world she has just entered, and you are trying to adjust to being a parent. We suggest that you cut yourself some slack and take some time to figure this whole sleeping business out. You are most likely going to make mistakes and have to adjust as you go along, as your needs change and as your baby's needs mature. While I was conducting research for this book, I did pretty much everything that the sleep experts tell you *not* to do, and both my son and I have survived!

As parents, we often have grandiose expectations when it comes to wanting a baby to sleep and getting our own sleep as parents. If you are the type of person who used to stay out all night partying and then effortlessly went to work in the morning, you'll be surprised to discover that a lack of sleep from parenting is FAR more exhausting. Remember that being responsive to your baby doesn't always mean picking her up, but it does mean acknowledging her needs. Don't ever get so overtired that you ignore or shut out your baby in an effort to catch some Z's, or you may break the trust you have built in your relationship. By now, you've probably figured out that your entire world has changed, whether you admit it or not, and you're going to have to decide if you need to shut off your cell phone, detach your door bell, or turn off the computer—because you just can't do it all. Some things will have to wait until both you and the baby have slept. E-mails and thank-you notes for baby gifts are not crucial during this bonding time, but sleep is.

Always have your pediatrician rule out any medical issues before following the recommended disciplines of any sleep experts. Medical conditions will always affect your baby's sleep cycles.

Sleep Schedules—Winding Down

Sleeping schedules are paramount for babies and children. We all know that sleep is an important part of development and of life, and it is up to the parents to try and implement a sleep schedule for their babies. Figure out a routine that works for you and your baby, with a goal of helping your baby go into a comfortable sleep mode. Maybe that could entail a warm bath after dinner, rocking the baby, and then putting her in her crib. Another option is feeding your baby and then taking her on a walk around the neighborhood to calm down before bed. Whatever you decide, stick to it, so your baby can start regulating her body and preparing for sleep.

Many parents worry that if they don't teach their babies to sleep correctly, they won't learn to soothe themselves and will encounter a lifetime of sleeping troubles. As you will learn, babies are resilient, and, like you, they can and will change. If your bedtime routine isn't working for you or your baby, you can always change it. It may take time, patience, and consistency, but it can change.

Most babies need help learning to soothe themselves back to sleep if they wake up briefly in the night, or they may take a bottle in the night or breastfeed. They may need to be rocked for a little bit, or perhaps have their back rubbed while they rest. If your child is still having difficulty calming down and you have swaddled her, rocked her, fed her, changed her, and you are out of ideas, make a loud "shushing" sound in her ear while gently moving her from side to side. This works a lot of the time, even for colicky babies. The "shushing" sound is similar to what your baby heard in the womb, as fluids moved around her. The side-to-side movement while holding her like a football moves the fluids in the inner ear, which is a calming rocking motion for her.

Beware that some soothing movements can be stimulating for your baby! Say what?! Indeed, some babies find rocking, patting, pacing, swinging, or even being picked up stimulating, and you may actually be creating an undesired effect on your baby. Instead of calming her, you may be waking her up and making her more alert. How can you tell? If your child is not getting tired, if she is flailing her limbs, or laughing, or getting more excited or even crying and thrashing, these are some of the signs your baby is being stimulated. You will have to change your approach. Maybe try calming music or apply deeper pressure with your fingertips, giving her more of a massage than a light pat. Try not to pick her up if she fusses, and just use a few reassuring murmurs, such as, "Mommy's here. Shhhh, shhhh." Some babies prefer less physical comforting and more auditory or visual security. Just knowing you're close by might be enough for your baby to soothe herself to sleep.

Sleeping Cues

How will you know if your baby is tired? Some sleep experts suggest writing down your baby's schedule (when she falls asleep and wakes up, when she eats and needs a diaper change) and watching your baby's behaviors and body language. Is she rubbing her eyes? Is she staring off into space? You want to try and learn your baby's cues, because there is nothing worse than an overtired baby cycle. It's like quicksand—once your baby is overtired, you will be spending all your time trying to get her back into a rested state, only it's hard for your baby to sleep when she's overly exhausted.

Baby's Body Clock

Yes, it does exist. While some sleep experts seem to think that all babies and humans have the same internal clock, we don't. According to John Medina, director of the Brain Center for Applied Learning Research at Seattle Pacific University and author of *Brain Rules,* some people are early risers, and some function best later in the day or in the early evening.[3] He divides these two groups into larks (early risers) and owls (late risers). I am an owl and was thrilled to have a child who is the same. We both love to go to sleep late and sleep in; however, my mother is a lark. She is up before the sun and has already cleaned the entire house before noon. How does this internal clock affect you and your baby? You may train your baby to sleep on certain cycles; however, you may always be battling his internal clock. Train your baby to sleep as much as possible, but also be flexible, taking into consideration whether he is an early riser or whether he likes to sleep the morning away.

Sleep Methods

There are many sleep methods, sleep specialists, and sleep books that you can explore to decide what is right for you and your baby. There are also some wonderful Web sites that have videos of sleep methods and examples other families have tried. We trust that you will find the best sleep method for you and your family.

Sensory Needs while Sleeping

Be open to and considerate of your baby's sensory needs. These needs may be disrupting your baby's sleep schedule. Does he need pressure to feel secure in his body? Did you stop swaddling too soon? Perhaps a sleep-positioner would help him to feel snuggled? Does your baby need a pacifier for sucking and calming? Does he need to be comforted to feel secure enough to sleep? Is he hungry? Are there crickets chirping outside the nursery? What is the baby's body temperature? Is he sweaty and hot, or clammy and cold? If you help your baby feel good, he will sleep better.

Where to Sleep?

You may choose to have your baby sleep in a crib, in a bassinet beside your bed, or in your bed. Whatever you choose, please make sure your baby is safe during the night in a secure, clutter-free area. Review our chapter on decorating the nursery for information about using a sensory-friendly crib.

If you sleep together in the same bed (which Jackie did), make sure your baby cannot fall off the bed. Use bedrails that are available online or at any Babies R Us. Also, make sure that you and your husband or partner do not roll over and smother the baby. If you're not a light sleeper or you drink alcohol or use medications, perhaps your baby should be close by in a crib. Always put your baby's safety first.

Sleep Patterns

When you first bring your baby home, his sleep patterns may be erratic. Within the first few weeks, as you get to know one another and each other's needs, you can decide what sleep schedule you'd like to adopt. Figuring out how to feed your baby, burp him, and dress him will exhaust you both, and hopefully you'll both be asleep in no time. Sounds easy, right? It can be, for some lucky families, and it can be very challenging for the rest of us.

It is recommended that newborns to infants 3 months old sleep 15 to 16 hours a day, give or take an hour. Often, babies can stay awake for 3 hours at a time and then sleep again. At 4 and 5 months of age, your baby may sleep a little less—between 14 and 15 hours—and will be able to stay awake for 3 $\frac{1}{2}$ hours at a time. Between 6 and 8 months, your baby should be sleeping 10 to 12 hours a night, sometimes waking in the middle of the night, and taking two to three naps during the day.

MOM TIP: *All the baby books I have read and all of the pediatricians I have spoken with confirm that babies sleep for most of their first year of life. That was not true in my case, as my son spent most of his first year wide awake. I know now that this was indicative of his SPD, but at the time, I just knew that something was wrong. Nothing could soothe my baby into sleep except pacing (back and forth for hours), bouncing on a ball, and nursing. Wow, was that first year tiring for me—but we got through it, and you and your baby will, too.*

We know of some rebellious parents who swear off routines and refuse to conform to a baby's sleep cycle. Their thought process is that the baby will adjust to their schedule. These parents refuse to acknowledge that their loud TV and brightly lit house affect their baby's sleep. We have heard them say things such as, "The baby will get used to it." These parents insist that a baby is supposed to adapt to their life, and not vice versa. It's such a strange concept to me as a mother to not want to fulfill my baby's needs, but we are all different. Hopefully, these parents have babies without sensory dysfunction, who will grow and prosper, regardless of their parents' inflexibility.

Keep in mind that the stages of a baby's growth pass quickly. You may be exhausted and overwhelmed right now, but soon, you'll be missing these glorious days of bonding with your baby. Take a deep breath and maybe a hot bath if you can, and steal some "you" time before taking on the nighttime routine if it's challenging for you and your baby.

Baby Naps

I just woke up, and you want me to go back to bed? Some babies will find it difficult to transition from being awake to playing and eating and then going back to sleep again, but keep at it. Before a nap, be sure to go through the "going to sleep routine" that you do in the evening, even if it is a modified and shorter routine. This will help your baby's body adjust back into sleep mode for naptime. These external clues will notify her internal system to prepare to nap.

Your baby should be more awake and alert during the day and should nap in the morning and afternoon. It is very important to have a schedule for your baby, so she can get enough sleep to be able to stay alert, play, and learn while she's awake. Make time for those naps, and if you need to, stay at home or make sure that your daycare provider or nanny sticks to a schedule. Consistency is still key during these heavy-sleep months.

Positioning Baby

Sleeping on the tummy versus on the back is always a hot topic. We typically tell families to have their baby sleep on her back (or side) to reduce the risk of Sudden Infant Death Syndrome, or SIDS. When babies begin to roll and are able to pick their heads up, they will be able to reposition themselves safely, and SIDS will not be as much of a concern. Some parents prefer to have their baby sleep on her side. Just make sure your pediatrician feels that sleeping on her side is medically safe for your baby. Make sure you still give your baby plenty of tummy time every day, since she will primarily be sleeping on her back. (See the next section for more information about tummy time.)

Are You Sleeping?

Between your lack of sleep and being constantly awakened by either your baby or your natural instinct to check on him, this time can be rough on new parents. Whether you are a working mom or a stay-at-home mom, if you are not sleeping, it may be dangerous. Be careful driving, operating machinery, and even carrying your baby around if you are truly exhausted. Without sleep, your brain cannot function at its full potential. If possible, ask your partner to take a night shift or two (maybe during the weekend) so that you can sleep yourself back to your natural state of mind. If you are a single parent, ask for help. Ask your mom or a friend to help you out.

Have you become a mom zombie? Are you angry with your baby for not sleeping? Do you have unrealistic expectations of your newborn because you have to get up and go to work in the morning? Are you at your wits' end because you have to get up and take your older children to school in a few hours, and your baby can't sleep? Our advice is to take a few moments to try to find your sense of inner peace. Go to that place of strength deep inside you, whether it be religious, spiritual, or biological. Find it, and breathe. Those old adages of counting to ten will actually make sense to you now. Breathe, and try to get some rest.

Here's some recommended reading if you're already awake at night:

- *The Baby Book,* by William Sears, Martha Sears, Robert Sears, and James Sears
- *The Baby Whisperer Solves All Your Problems,* by Tracy Hogg and Melinda Blau
- *The Happiest Baby on the Block: The New Way to Calm Crying and Help Your Newborn Sleep Longer,* by Harvey Karp
- *The Sleep Lady's Good Night, Sleep Tight,* by Kim West, LCSW-C, with Joanne Kenen

The Importance of Tummy Time

OCCUPATIONAL THERAPIST TIP: *From a sensory and development perspective, begin with "tummy time" as soon as you get home from the hospital. A few minutes a day with supervision will really strengthen your baby's head and neck muscles, and he will begin holding his head up after the first couple of weeks. This developmental position is crucial for your baby's development of motor skills, as well as increasing the tactile awareness of your baby's cheeks, which helps with oral-motor skills.*

Tummy time is when your baby lays on his stomach, on a blanket or a baby-friendly mat placed on the floor or on a table with supervision. Always stay with your baby during tummy time and lower yourself to be at eye level with them. Talk to your baby, sing to him, or be silly to encourage your baby to lift his head. You can also have "tummy-to-tummy" time with your baby. Start by leaning back at a 45° angle, on either the couch or the floor, making sure your back is securely supported (with pillows or the like). Next, place your baby onto your chest, on his tummy. He will be on his stomach, but able to look up at you. You may also try this while you are lying flat.

When you place a child on his stomach, he usually does not like having his face down in the carpet, or he is interested in the fun baby mat he's lying on, so he will eventually learn to turn his head from side to side and to lift it up off the floor. Be patient. This make take some time and practice. If your baby gets a little fussy on his tummy, that's okay. If he's crying uncontrollably, he may have reflux or an upset tummy. Move him to a more comfortable position, and try "tummy time" later.

If your baby seems to be really struggling with tummy time, there are items on the market to get your baby off the ground, such as the Learning Curve Winnie the Pooh Tummy Time Garden Spin. This allows your baby to be on his tummy, while elevated with support. Your baby then gets to spin himself around by using his arm muscles, which is good for babies who may be a little delayed in their floor mobility. We don't recommend that you rely on these props for too long, as you want your baby to build more and more strength by pushing up his body weight, but these devices may get him started.

Many babies love "tummy time." First, they learn to pick their heads up and then push up on their hands. Next, they will get strong enough to reach out for a toy with one hand, while they bear weight on the other hand. Once your baby is comfortable, she will really want to get off her tummy, so she will turn her head to one side, performing what is called an *asymmetrical tonic neck reflex*, with one arm tucked under her body and the other arm out to the side where her face is turned.

She will then swing that arm over and roll to her side and then onto her back! Ta-dah! She has learned to roll! Congratulations, baby!

It's exciting to babies to know that they can be on their tummies and, when they want to turn over and look at something different, they can roll. While they are lying on their backs and they see something they want that is out of reach, they will eventually learn to swing that arm across their bodies and roll onto the side and then onto their tummies. Now they can push up, look around, and reach out for that toy. All the while, they are strengthening their core (tummy) muscles and their arms and legs. Soon they will learn to push up to all four limbs on their hands and knees.

Before long, your baby will begin to rock back and forth on his hands and knees and eventually begin moving forward and/or crawling. Some babies do what is called an "army crawl," where their stomachs touch the ground and they pull themselves by their arms, pushing slightly forward with their feet. This is okay for them to do, but you still want to encourage a full crawling position. Some babies do learn all of these skills, but not necessarily in this order. Some babies stand and cruise before they ever crawl; some babies only commando or army crawl, and some babies scoot on their bottoms. All of these movements promote movement and learning, which is a good thing.

Play

Play is an integral part of childhood development. As humans, we use play to connect and reconnect after being away from each other, to explore our environment, to learn how to behave, and to learn how to complete ordinary life tasks. Play is used to help us cope, survive, and interact with the world. It opens the door of the imagination, allowing our creativity to flow through us.

The crib is for your baby to sleep in; therefore, she doesn't necessarily need to be playing in there. It is helpful if you have a designated area for her to play in, whether that is a Pack 'n Play (a playpen) or a place on the floor that has been baby proofed. It is important to hold your baby and carry her close to you, but it is equally important to allow your child to move on the floor and develop her motor skills. Put her down and watch her learn through her natural environment.

Play "Peek-a-boo" with your baby. Mirroring (imitating) your baby and having her imitate you can be a fun way to bond and learn. Stick your tongue out at your baby and see if she copies your actions. Rattles are exciting for babies. Move them, and they make noise! It can be very powerful for a little one to embrace this cause and effect at her command. If you really want to entertain your baby, be a magician. Show your baby a toy, then hide it behind your back. The toy is gone. Then it reappears. This may seem simple to us, but it will bring great delight to a baby who is learning about her external world.

There are a number of toys you can pick out for your baby. Some have lights, some have music, and some are an entire sensory entertainment unit in one. Monitor your baby and make sure that these fantastic items are not overwhelming or overstimulating your little one.

Signs that your baby may have sensory sensitivities or is overloaded:

- While trying to play with your baby, she stiffens or arches her back to get away from you.
- She turns her head away and averts her eyes from you while you are trying to engage her in play.
- She prefers to play alone and stares down at her feet to calm herself.

Neuroscientists have confirmed that your baby's sensory systems are being hardwired during the first few years of life.[4] It is up to you as a parent to provide your baby with an appropriate learning environment. No pressure, right? It is really about providing enough stimulation and variety to your baby's brain to encourage growth and development. This does not ensure that there won't be complications, but by playing with your baby and being aware of her behaviors, you may discover any concerns at an early age, and we'll help point you in the right direction for treatment.

What are some of the items in your baby's world? Does he have a gurgling aquarium hanging in his crib? Does your baby enjoy watching the plastic fish swim back and forth? How can you tell? If he is kicking his legs and watching the aquarium, chances are he's enjoying it. If he is turning away and fussing, it's a safe bet that he would like you to turn the gurgling off. Watch your baby for cues.

Hanging mobiles are great for newborns, who can see motion better than still objects. As he tries to focus on a swinging bug, he's building the basic elements of visual perception. It may seem as though your baby is just lying there watching a mobile, but he's also developing the ability to detect colors, edges, contrast, and shapes.

While your baby may have many objects to look at and play with, the most engaging toy is YOU. Your baby innately desires to interact with you and his other family members. So have fun playing with your baby—this time will pass quickly!

Developmentally Appropriate Toys: 0 to 6 Months

These are just suggestions we like to give parents and families that will encourage cognitive, motor, visual, and social development in your infant.

- *Any sort of rattle or toy that babies can shake back and forth.* Rattles help develop a baby's auditory system, while she is also learning proprioception (where her hand is) and how to control her swinging arm.

- *Rings to hold onto, and toys that are soft and safe to put in the mouth.* Your baby is working on her grasp and feeling different textures.

- *Any sort of nontoxic teething toy* (The First Years vibrating star teether is a favorite).

- *Cause-and-effect toys.* For example, when your baby pushes a button that makes Oscar the Grouch pop out of his trash can, she starts to make the connection that the button will always make Oscar appear.

- *Hand-eye coordination toys.* Shape sorters and ring stackers are always good as baby learns about shapes and how to control her hands.

- *Any and every BABY book!* READ TO YOUR CHILD! (*Note:* The soft plush books are nice, and the cardboard ones are more durable for use with babies.)

- *Baby-safe mirrors are fun.* What could be better than looking at their own sweet faces? This helps with visual perception and building self-confidence.

- *Toys that play nursery rhymes or ABC songs* (Munchkin Mozart Magic Cube is a personal favorite). They stimulate the auditory system and help teach cause and effect.

Developmental Milestones, 0 to 6 Months

Babies develop at different rates and accomplish various milestones at different times, so please don't worry if your child is not exactly on track. We will tell you what signs you should be looking for—if there is a delay, you can talk to your pediatrician, but again—EVERY child is different. That is what makes us so wonderful as human beings!

1-2 MONTHS

Gross- and Fine-Motor Development
- Displays jerky hand and arm movements
- Brings one hand to his mouth, hands are fists
- Lifts his head while lying on his tummy
- Moves his head side to side while lying on his tummy
- Brings his hands to midline while lying on his back

Visual Development
- Can focus 8-12 inches from his face
- Sees better in black or white or in highly contrasting colors
- Prefers to look a at human face, especially his mother's face
- Follows a moving person with his eyes while lying on his back
- Has fully developed hearing

Touch and Smell Development
- Recognizes the smell of mother's breast milk
- Prefers sweeter smells
- Prefers gentle touch rather than course touch

Speech and Language Development
- Startles at loud sounds
- Quiets when spoken to
- Makes cooing sounds

Social/Cognitive Development

- Smiles as a reflex
- Establishes eye contact
- Begins to draw attention to himself when he is distressed
- May begin to suck on his fingers at 1-4 months

Things to look out for at 1 month

- Stiffness or not moving the arms and legs much
- Poor suck or swallow or not gaining weight—check with your pediatrician about how much your baby should be gaining
- Not blinking at a bright light
- Not responding to loud sounds

3-4 MONTHS

Gross- and Fine-Motor Development

- Should be able to pick her head up when lying on her stomach
- Should be able to stretch out her legs and kick when lying on her back
- Grasps and shakes hand toys
- Begins to roll from her back to her tummy
- Holds her head up in supported sitting
- Opens her hands up more and brings them to midline
- Clasps her hands and grasps her toys actively

Visual-Motor Development

- Picks up small objects or toys
- Hits dangling objects, like those on a mobile
- Manipulates objects in her hands

Speech and Language Development

- Seems to recognize her mother's voice
- Cries differently for different needs
- Smiles when she sees you

- Watches your face when you speak
- Makes noises when talked to

Social/Cognitive Development

- Socializes with strangers
- Stops unexplained crying
- Can tell the difference between mommy and a stranger
- Enjoys social play, like "Peek-a-boo"
- Recognizes her bottle visually
- May begin to eat pureed foods and/or rice cereal—check with your pediatrician on when to start baby foods
- Begins putting her hands up to her bottle

5-6 MONTHS

Gross- and Fine-Motor Development

- Is able to move his head side to side while sitting
- Sits by leaning on hands
- Can almost bear his entire weight on his legs
- Pulls clothing over his face
- Opens hands more and the fingers straighten out
- Reaches for and grasps objects
- Can drop and pick up a toy
- Bangs objects on a table
- Transfers an object from one hand to the other
- Holds his own bottle
- May push up to all fours from his tummy
- May begin to rock back and forth on his hands and knees
- Lunges forward and reaches while in a sitting position without losing his balance

Speech and Language Development

- Responds to changes in the tone of your voice
- Notices that toys make sounds
- Vocalizes excitement and displeasure
- Makes gurgling sounds

Social/Cognitive Development

- Lifts his arms to be picked up
- May start displaying some stranger anxiety (or may not until 7-8 months)
- Explores adults' facial features and hand features
- Recognizes his own name
- Displays stranger anxiety
- Enjoys social play
- Explores his hands and mouth
- Is interested in mirror images
- Opens his mouth when presented with food on a spoon
- Eats fruits and vegetables and gums dissolvable foods

If your child is not on target with her developmental milestones and you are concerned, consult with your pediatrician. Many times, as an occupational therapist, I have parents bring their kids in for occupational therapy around 1 or 2 years of age, and I ask them why they waited so long to come see me. The parents will many times reply that their doctor told them to wait and see. Well, sometimes that is the best thing to do, but other times it is not.

Speech therapist Nicole Collings states, *"It does not hurt to at least have an evaluation completed by a therapist if you are concerned about your child, but it CAN hurt to wait!"*

CHAPTER THREE

Baby Life
(6 Months to 1 Year)

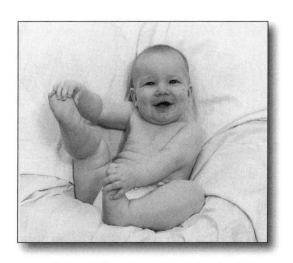

He was always grabbing his feet!
ODIN, 6 MONTHS OLD

Rolling Over, Sitting Up, and Reaching

Rolling Over

SINCE EVERY CHILD DEVELOPS AT DIFFERENT LEVELS, WE WILL DESCRIBE SOME ways to encourage your baby to work on rolling, sitting, and reaching. Most babies have been lying on their tummies since birth and have good head control as they lift their heads while on their tummies. They will then begin to push up on their arms and support their weight with their arms. When trying to roll, usually the baby will get a little frustrated from being on her tummy and want to move, so she exhibits an asymmetrical tonic neck reflex, where one arm is bent and other reaches out straight. With the straight arm, she swings it around as she brings her head in that direction and rolls from her tummy to her back. If your baby is having difficulty rolling and she is already more than 4 months of age, you may want to practice having her lie on her side and then use a toy to encourage her to flip over onto her back. Then you can progress to having her reach out her arm while she's on her tummy and help her roll over. Eventually, most babies learn this on their own, but you can always encourage them to play on the floor and use toys to motivate them to want to roll over.

Sitting

By 6 months, your baby should already have good head control, and when you hold him under his arms, he can turn his head from side to side. You can help him sit up by propping pillows behind him or by holding him in a sitting position to help strengthen his tummy muscles. Some parents choose to sit their babies in what's called a Bumbo chair. This can be nice to help contain the baby briefly while you are doing something else, or you can place a toy on the tray for the baby to play with, but this Bumbo chair is not going to engage the "sitting up" muscles. You have to actually work with him and help him to sit up on the floor first, until he can do it on his own. When babies are sitting on the floor and you are either supporting them or they have pillows propped around them, they will activate their abdominal muscles to stay upright. Make sure you have him on a carpet or a soft blanket and sit with your baby, in case he tips over. It's okay for him to gently fall, but you don't want him to hit his head on the ground. Once he is able to sit independently, he will then begin to reach for toys and play with them while he sits up. This is called *dynamic sitting,* and it works his core muscles, which he will need for crawling, walking, and other types of movement.

As your baby grows stronger and stronger, she will get ready to transition from a sitting position to a crawling or tummy position. You can encourage your baby to sit, and then put a toy just out of reach so she has to lean forward and move her body from sitting to either all fours or her tummy so she can reach the toy. These are the beginning steps for crawling. Don't worry if your child is not crawling by 6 months of age—some babies crawl at 9 months or even later.

Reaching

Your baby has been reaching and grasping for months, but around 6 months or so, his reaching will be more controlled. Now you will notice your baby manipulating his fingers and thumbs and becoming more accurate with his movements. He will work toward developing a pincer grasp (which is how we pick up items with our fingers and thumbs). For example, your baby may be able to pick up your car keys and hold onto them. Interestingly enough, it is harder for your baby to release this grasp, a skill that comes later. Remember that your child is depending on his vision at this point to see items that he's reaching for. As his sight improves, so will his reaching. He also has to *want* to reach an item. So keep those toys just a little way away from your baby so he gets a workout as he goes for it.

Crawling—Motor Planning

We cannot stress enough how important it is in motor development and overall development to have your baby crawl. Encourage her to do this by starting tummy time early, so she will enjoy or tolerate being on her stomach. Once she starts pushing up to her hands and knees and rocking back and forth, put her toy just out of reach so she has to move to get it. Some babies pick up crawling quickly, and others take a little while to get the hang of it.

Do not let your baby skip this milestone if she prefers to be upright. While the verdict is still out on the importance of crawling, just remember that your baby's brain is being wired at this time. Some experts have pointed out that crawling stimulates the same areas of the brain as those used to learn to read and write. These parts of the brain also control speech.

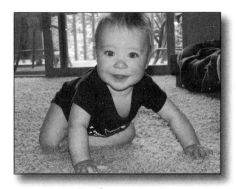

On the goooooo!
CAIUS AT 6 MONTHS

Crawling is the first step in learning how to use both sides of the body in bilateral coordination and in reciprocal movements. When learning to crawl, you are exhibiting your symmetrical tonic neck reflex. This means that if your arms and neck are extended, your legs are flexed, and when your neck begins to flex, your arms flex and your legs extend, which moves you forward in a crawling or walking motion.

Learning to crawl sets a foundation for problem-solving skills because the baby will need to figure out how to get to that desired toy by moving to where the toy is. You don't have to get your baby so worked up that he screams every time you encourage him to crawl, but practice a little bit each day until he gets the hang of it. If he is not catching on, give him some more time. If he is not crawling by 10 months of age, you might ask your pediatrician about it.

Again, on the flip side, some pediatricians do not see any significance in crawling whatsoever. From an occupational therapist and a mom's perspective, it is our preference to encourage crawling.

Activities and Technology

While not everything is good for your baby, it's not all bad, either. We're not antitechnology or antitelevision. You cannot keep your baby in a bubble, but at the same time, it's up to you to pick the right things for your baby and to not rely on the Disney Channel to be your full-time babysitter. What's a happy medium? Well, you have a lot to choose from these days, and making a choice can be overwhelming. Don't try to do it all. Your baby does not need to know HTML or learn second languages, sign language, math, and reading before 6 months of age, but you can pick one of these academic pursuits and use it to spend quality time with your child.

Just remember, some babies will not enjoy being drilled with flash cards, and others will enjoy the attention and praise they receive. If you feel that it's important to begin teaching your child these skills at such a young age, you might ask yourself why. Do you think this will make him smarter? Do you feel that it will give him an advantage later in life? Or are you doing it to satisfy your own ego? We think you should let your baby be a baby. Take him on a walk and show him the trees and flowers. Enjoy this time with your child—it will go by fast. Forcing your child to learn computer code will not make him the next Bill Gates multibillionaire mogul.

Here are some examples of what is on the market, but we would like to emphasize that we still recommend a walk in the park over a television show, a DVD, or flash cards any day of the week (and we have put out our own set of DVDs!). We'll also talk about classes you and your baby can take and how this aids in his development.

Television

Babies and toddlers now have dedicated channels to choose from—Sprout, Noggin, and PBS, to name a few. While the programming is usually educational and entertaining, watch with your child and make sure that the shows you're picking are packed with ideas and images that you want going into her brain. For example, "Sesame Street" is a classic favorite, but understand that political groups, food groups, and vaccination groups may pay for advertising that is built into the show. Make sure your child's brain is being pumped with information that you agree with and foods that you want her to eat. For example, if a show pushes milk, and you're a dairy-free family, you don't have to watch that show. There are many to choose from.

What is a good amount of television to watch? While there is no perfect answer, we say, "not too much." We have done some research, and everyone has a different opinion. The American Academy of Pediatrics says that you shouldn't allow your child to watch TV until after 2 years of age because it can negatively affect early brain development. Others say no TV in the first 12 months of life. We say, ultimately, it's the parents' choice, and we want you to be an involved parent. It's just as easy to put your child in a playpen with some toys while you take a shower or wash dishes as it is to sit him in the Bumbo chair or a swing to watch TV. If you do allow your child to watch some shows, limit the time, depending on how old he is, and make sure the show is age appropriate for your child to encourage learning. Please refer to the American Academy of Pediatrics for a guideline for the amount of TV your child should watch. The younger the child, the less he should watch (if any at all).

Commercials can be a culprit in your child's troublesome behavior down the road. Messages about toys and the latest crazes are foisted mercilessly on their formative brains, which can turn a quick trip to the store into a full-fledged tantrum standoff. Children don't understand that they won't die without these items after being drilled that they need to have the latest and greatest. When you're doing battle in the grocery-store line, you may realize that perhaps letting your child watch hours of TV and commercials wasn't such a good idea after all. With today's technology, you can always use Tivo or DVR to record shows and remove commercials entirely. It won't end tantrums, but it may help curb your child's appetite for some highly marketed items.

- *Baby Bumblebee DVDs.* This DVD series is popular in the special-needs community, but it's good for typically developing children, as well. What I like about this series is that it's repetitive and basic. My son loved these DVDs, as he was trying to catch up with the development level of other toddlers—but they might not keep a typically developing child's attention for long. They focus on vocabulary and word groups, such as actions, opposites, and questions.

- *Baby Einstein DVDs.* Unless I'm mistaken, these videos do not proclaim to make your child a genius like Einstein. The classical music is delightful for adults and for baby. The puppets are fun, and there is enough activity to keep your baby engaged for 24 minutes while Mommy showers or Daddy makes dinner. The fact that Disney bought this franchise and expanded on it confirms that this is entertainment and not baby brain-cell fertilizer. These DVDs are fun, clean, engaging entertainment for baby. My son loved these videos, and I knew that I could jump in the shower, brush my teeth, and get dressed in the duration of one show.

- *Baby Sign-Language DVDs.* There are a few DVD series to choose from. "Signing Time" is popular and was featured on PBS. The theory is that motor skills develop before verbal skills, and, therefore, your child will be less frustrated and better able to communicate before she's able to speak. Britt encourages signing, knowing that babies are able to start signing around 9 months. Parents should start signing with their baby at 6 months, using verbal cues as well as hand gestures. See section D of this chapter, Teaching Your Baby Sign Language, for more details. Friends of mine who have tried signing with their babies have had mixed results. The ones that have been successful and consistent and who continue to use sign language and hand signals into their child's formative years swear by it. One friend was the envy of all of us—her child would look to her for a signal before crossing the street, while the rest of us were screaming at our children. They had almost a secret language and could communicate from across the room. Other moms who have tried sign language didn't take into account that they would have to learn to sign as well, and they didn't want to put the time or effort into learning it. With my son's sensory issues and my lack of sleep, I didn't even consider taking on a new language.

- *Baby Learns a Second Language.* Little Pim is a popular brand of DVDs that teaches foreign languages to children. If you are from another country or if you and your family speak a second language, these are fantastic visual and audio tools to help your baby learn. For those of you who speak one language, these are a fun way for your baby to be exposed to other languages and cultures, but we're not sure how much he will remember, unless the language learning is consistent and reinforced throughout childhood and into adulthood. Another plus would be if your family has adopted a child from another country and you'd like him to learn his native tongue, or if you'd like your child to learn some Hebrew for religious purposes. One suggestion for families who are bilingual is to have the mom speak only Spanish to the child, for instance, and to have the dad speak only English to the child, starting from the time he is born. This can help the child learn both languages. Before the age of 7 is when it is easiest to learn new languages in addition to your native language, so this is the time to teach your children. If you are not bilingual, you can have them take classes as they get older and begin doing school-age activities. Again, pick and choose what works best for your family and don't try to prepare your child for college in his infancy.

- *Hooked on Phonics.* This series provides valuable tools for age-appropriate learning that will translate into what your child is learning in the school system. One complaint I hear about teaching a baby to read is many programs focus on entire-word memorization, rather than sounding words out. Hooked on Phonics does this. They have games, and they make learning fun with a reward system of stickers as your child accomplishes levels. The program now starts with a 3-month-old level, but moms, if you wait until your child is preparing for preschool or kindergarten, your child will learn to read in ample time to graduate from high school. They also have math programs, as well as a selection of languages to choose from.

Of note, some research states that a child's brain development does not facilitate understanding how to read until the age of 5 or 6 years, and if we try to push reading too early, then it only makes things more difficult down the road.[5] We really shouldn't be trying to teach our children to read and write until their brains are truly ready. Children have to have fully developed sensory systems to be able to utilize all the correct components to do such demanding tasks. Let your baby be a baby, and focus on gross-motor development first. The rest will follow.

Social Classes for Your Baby

While you can take your baby for playdates in the park and to your friends' and families' homes, there are also structured playgroups available to you and your baby. These can be helpful if you're not comfortable facilitating play with your baby and would like ideas and guidance or if you just want to expose your baby to music and other social environments. It's good for Mom and Dad to get out of the house and socialize with other parents, too.

If your baby is not having fun at one of these locations and is over-stimulated or fussy, take a break from going, and try again when your baby is older. I tried to take my son to a social group with music, imaginative climbing structures, and play, and he arched his back and howled in pain at the mere suggestion of circle time. Since he was hypersensitive, these groups were too much for him and caused him mental and physical distress. Taking him to these classes actually provided an excellent (yet heart-wrenching) environment in which to view how sensitive he really was and persuaded me that he did need help with his sensory systems. If your baby has this reaction, skip to chapter 7, where we discuss children who may have sensory-processing difficulties.

- *Gymboree.* Gymboree offers play and music classes for babies and toddlers. These can be a fun way for your child to get to make noise with musical instruments, and you don't have to have them in your home if the noise bothers you. A parent or caregiver participates with the child, which is a good way to share a special experience with him without having to do all the work yourself. These gyms are usually bright, colorful, and attractive, with climbing activities and playground equipment that encourage motor-skills development and organization of behavior. Your child's sensory systems will definitely get a workout at these joints.

- *Mommy & Me.* There is Mommy & Me everything! Yoga, play groups, art class, music—everything under the sun. Mommy & Me has created an awesome brand that encourages Mommy to get out there, share her baby with the world, and enjoy time with her. Often, new moms can feel isolated and confined to a baby's schedule and world, especially if they don't have friends or family close by with a baby. Mommy & Me and other similar classes and brands offer moms outlets and a chance for social interaction with other moms like themselves. Many of their activities encourage sensory development, such as yoga. We're big proponents of the ancient tradition of yoga, as it builds strength while calming the body.

Baby Yoga

Parents can do yoga with their babies starting around 6 months of age, and some places start even younger than that. There are many different books and Web sites that offer poses and techniques. Sites that I recommend to families I work with are *www.yogababies.co.uk* and *www.sweetpeayoga.com.* Check your local yoga studio and see what they have to offer in the way of classes for your infant or toddler. Yoga can be a good way to bond with your baby, stretch her out, and help her learn to self-soothe and regulate herself, as well as give you some relaxation. Plus, it's fun!

Indoor Playgrounds

Thankfully, there are indoor playgrounds babies and toddlers can explore and socialize in, even when the weather doesn't permit you to go outside. If you and your baby are feeling cooped up and adventurous, look for a local indoor playground. While they may be a breeding ground for germs, most of these places follow strict guidelines for cleanliness and sanitation. If your child has allergies or asthma, ask which cleaning products they use and make sure the rooms are well ventilated. Another good thing about these indoor playgrounds is that there are rules. Unlike outdoor public parks, rules are enforced, and kids are not permitted to get too rowdy and wild. Remember that these playgrounds can cause sensory overload and meltdowns, so watch your child to make sure he is having fun. It's time to leave if you see signs that he is getting tired, hungry, or overstimulated.

Teaching Your Baby Sign Language

Using sign language increases verbal language abilities, and we personally believe that every baby can benefit from learning some simple baby signs. Even if your child's hearing is normal, sign language is a way for babies to communicate before they can actually say words. We suggest that you start to teach your baby sign language as early as 6 months of age. Some moms start with their babies at birth, but since a baby doesn't have the motor skills to imitate any signs yet, by the time they are 6 months old, they may be burnt out.

Work on some simple baby signs that your baby can use to communicate her needs. You do not need to learn American Sign Language if your child is not hearing impaired. You can search out basic baby signs and even make up some that your baby does on her own, as long as you both understand what it means when she uses the sign.

Signing is EASY! There are simple books on baby signs, and you can always search the Internet for suggestions. Some of our favorites are *www.sign2me.com* and *Baby Signs,* by Joy Allen. However, we recommend any baby sign-language book that can help you (as a parent) learn.

Here are some signs you might begin working on with your baby:

- Milk
- Eat
- Play
- Sleep
- Animal signs (cat, dog, pig, etc)
- Mommy
- Daddy

Many people make the mistake of teaching their child to use the sign "More," but they don't pair the sign with any words or other signs. Then your toddler is signing "More" to you and crying, because you have no idea what she wants more of! I always tell the families that I work with to pair the sign for "More" with another word, like "Eat" or "Milk." Then your child learns to sign the word she actually means and can pair two signs together later. "More" is very easy for babies to pick up on, but you can just as easily teach them the actual sign for what they want.

Play

We asked occupational therapist Aviva Weiss for her expert advice on play. She not only works in pediatrics, but she is the mother of five children under the age of 9! We agreed that she, of anyone we could hit up, has both the personal and the professional experience to guide us.

- *Which toys do you feel are best for a child's sensory and developmental growth?*

  The best toys engage a child to move, think, and imagine on her own. These do not need to be expensive or technology-driven or overly complicated—just well made, fun, and colorful.

- *How many times a day do you recommend for parents to play with their children?*

  The optimal frequency depends on a child's age. Newborns and infants need constant play experiences in the form of sensory stimulation, including touch, visual and auditory stimulation, and movement. Babies should be engaged and responded to regularly throughout the day, not just when they cry. Talking and singing, rocking, and cuddling are all critical for infant development.

  In general, I recommend for a parent to interact with a child continually, whether it be making eye contact when the child talks or giving direct responses to show that the parent is listening and available to meet the needs of the child. Physical contact is also crucial. Children need to feel warm touches every day, whether they are hugs and kisses, a high five, or a reassuring pat on the back. I also believe that a parent should spend at least 10 minutes each day engaging in a child-driven activity. This builds and enhances the relationship between parent and child and reinforces the child's awareness of his own abilities and interests.

- *What are the most important types of play for a child?*

  Play should engage all the senses and enable the child to be an active participant. The types of play will vary, depending on age and the child's stage of development. Play through exploration—touching, feeling, moving, and tasting—is crucial for the development of a small baby and toddler. Active play is consistently important throughout childhood, as crawling, running, jumping, cycling, climbing, and participating in sports strengthens the body and develops the mind. As a child reaches the age of 3, pretend play becomes crucial to the developing awareness of relationships and his role in the greater picture of life. As logic (ages 4-7) and more complex reasoning kicks in (ages 7-12), games that develop logic and cognition are great.

  In general, combining different play experiences develops a child's motor strength, cognition, awareness of self in relation to others, self-esteem, and social skills. Think of it as having a "balanced" toy chest, so even if your child favors building blocks and toys he can ride on (such as scooters and bikes), for example, he still has access to puzzles, books, crafts, and dress-up materials.

- *For parents of children with SPD, what are the top five pieces of therapy equipment that parents should talk to their occupational therapist about and consider investing in?*

  Each child has different needs, but some of the very helpful and popular choices for SPD are:
  - Tactile tummy and saddle scooters
  - Therapy/exercise balls and peanut balls
  - Trampoline
  - Swing (to hang inside the house)

– Weighted or compression vest, shirt, hat, and other clothing

- *What would you like to say to parents who may be raising typically developing children as well as children with special needs and/or SPD?*

  All children need love and *structure,* whether they have special needs or not. Talk to your children, take interest in their interests, and help them know and develop their talents and passions. Try to spend at least 10 minutes of private time with each child every day. Remember the big picture: It's all about helping your child develop into an emotionally healthy adult, to the best of her ability. And, it's normal to stumble from time to time. You can do it!

About Aviva Weiss, MS, OTR/L

Aviva Weiss MS, OTR/L, is the president and cofounder of Fun and Function, LLC, *(www.funandfunction.com)* and By Kids Only *(www.by kidsonly.com).* These companies are revolutionizing the way children face challenges while integrating more effectively into mainstream life. Founded in 2005, Fun and Function designs versatile toys, games, and therapy products that help all children realize their full potential, especially those with specific developmental needs.

A pediatric occupational therapist by vocation, Weiss was inspired to launch Fun and Function when she observed her infant daughter exhibiting sensory-processing difficulties, a condition marked by motor-coordination challenges and hypersensitivity to certain sensory stimuli. To help her daughter, Weiss shopped for a therapeutic weighted vest, known for its soothing effects, but was unable to find an attractive one at any price. She began to design her own, which led to a full line of toys, equipment, and costumes.

Prior to founding Fun and Function, she worked at leading institutions, including the Children's Hospital of Philadelphia and St Christopher's Hospital. She earned her bachelor's degree in psychology from Touro College and her master's degree in occupational therapy from The Richard Stockton College.

Developmentally Appropriate Toys: 6 to 12 Months

- Books, books, and more books! Anything colorful and interactive, where your baby has to lift things and open flaps, is good for him. READ TO YOUR BABY!
- Ring stackers, shape sorters, and cause-and-effect toys
- Fun bath toys, water squirters, and bath crayons for 10-12 months and older
- Toys for making music, tambourines, and pianos
- Blocks for building
- Toys that vibrate when you pull a string
- Any safe teething toy (Baby Einstein Teeth and Tug Pal are popular)
- Toys with various textures to them, such as beanbags made with different fabrics
- Puzzles with large wooden pieces and large wooden knobs for your baby to grasp
- Stuffed animals and toys she can begin pretend play with around 10-12 months

This list could truly go on forever. When picking out a toy, remember to avoid any small parts that your baby can put in her mouth and choke on. Read the toy labels to locate the recommended age group. Think of toys that will encourage your baby to interact with the toy and also with you. We are big believers in interactive, educational toys, because toys are fun, and they stimulate your baby's sensory systems, developmental growth, and curiosity. Whether they're store-bought toys or household items, your baby is developing his fine-motor and gross-motor skills and learning about our world. Most things are interesting to your baby, especially your keys and cell phone!

6-7 MONTHS

Gross- and Fine-Motor Development
- Lifts her head when pulled into a sitting position
- Rolls from her back to her tummy
- Bears some weight on her legs and bounces up and down on her feet
- Sits independently and may use her hands to play in a sitting position
- Starts leaning forward and moving from a sitting position down to her tummy
- Keeps her hands open most of the time
- Manipulates toys
- Bangs a toy on the table

Visual Development
- Feeds herself finger foods
- Drops small objects into a small cup

Speech and Language Development
- Enjoys Peek-a-boo games
- Turns and looks in the direction of sounds
- Pays attention to music

Social and Cognitive Development
- Smiles at herself in the mirror
- Shows anxiety when separating from her mother
- Bites food
- Bites and chews on toys

8-9 MONTHS

Gross- and Fine-Motor Development
- Crawls backwards
- Rocks back and forth on her hands and knees
- Crawls forward
- Makes stepping movements when you hold her hands
- Moves into a sitting position without help
- Stands when holding onto something
- Lets go of objects on purpose
- Can bang two blocks together
- Rakes her hand across small pieces (like Cheerios) to pick them up

Speech and Language Development
- Recognizes some familiar words (ie, milk, mommy, shoe)
- Tries to repeat sounds she hears from other adults
- Tries to communicate via actions or gestures
- Babbles short and long sounds

Social and Cognitive Development
- Shows a like or dislike for certain people and objects
- May start getting clingy with her mother
- Drools less, except when teething
- Reaches for small objects with one hand

10-12 MONTHS

Gross- and Fine-Motor Development
- May begin taking steps
- Cruises around furniture
- Lowers herself onto the floor from a standing position when holding onto something
- Stands independently for a few seconds before losing her balance
- Begins poking at things with her pointer finger

- Puts objects into a container
- Drinks from a sippy cup
- Uses a pincer grasp (thumb and pointer finger) to pick up small objects

Speech and Language Development

- Begins to respond to requests (eg, "Want more?" or "Come here.")
- Imitates different speech sounds
- Can say one or two words (bye-bye, dada, mama), although they may not be clear or she may not understand what it means
- Attends to a book or toy for 1-2 minutes
- Recognizes her own name

Social and Cognitive Development

- Holds a spoon
- Finger-feeds herself
- Tries to help with dressing by extending one arm through a shirt sleeve
- Eats most foods while using a munching pattern to chew

Toddler Time
(1 to 2 Years)

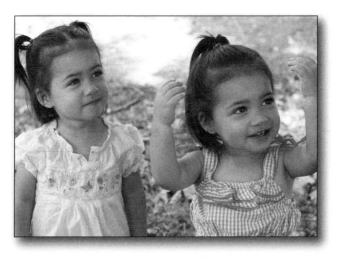

Twins are so lucky, they have a best friend at birth!
MIA AND ALLISON (ONE YEAR OLD)

Baby Learns to Walk

As an occupational therapist, I don't recommend using a walker for your baby as the only source of helping him learn to walk. These can be a fall risk, and it is better to have your child learn to crawl, stand, cruise, and then walk at his own pace. That said, falling is something that every child will do, and by falling, they learn about their body awareness and space. Sometimes when they use a walker toy, babies get dependent on them and it takes longer for them to learn to walk on their own.

After learning to crawl, babies tend to pull themselves up to a standing position and then begin to take steps while holding onto furniture to keep them steady. Next they will want to hold an adult's hand and take steps, placing their feet one in front of the other. Some babies will pull to a stand, cruise to another piece of furniture, stand alone, and then drop to a sit or crawling position and crawl to where they want to go. Eventually, when they are ready, they will begin taking steps. They will do this in their own time.

In Due Time

So many times I see families who encourage their child to walk early. One kiddo comes to mind who was an early crawler and stood up early. Everyone got so excited that he was standing at around 9 months old, and they wanted him to walk. If the baby is ready, he will do it—you cannot force the child to do something that his mind and development are not ready for. This particular child continued to crawl and pull himself up, then began to cruise and eventually walked right around 12 months of age, which is right on target. You don't have to have the fastest, smartest best baby on the block. Sometimes, he needs time to develop all the skills involved before taking off.

NOTE: Typically, boys are stronger motorically, and girls are stronger with language skills, so don't be alarmed if your second child is a girl and is not walking at the same time as your boy did. The typical age for starting to walk can be any time from 9 months to 14 months. You should not really begin to worry unless your child is not walking around 16 months of age.

Mommy's and Daddy's Backs

For quite some time, you've used your muscles to carry your baby around, and now you find yourself hunched over, holding your baby's hands as she masters walking. Try to bend at the knees and keep your shoulders back to avoid soreness. Your baby is going to be delighted to be mastering this milestone, and she's entering into an entirely new phase of freedom. Know that while you're aiding your baby in walking, she's building strength and developing her balance and posture. She will be an independent walker once her motor and sensory systems are ready.

Baby on the Move

You're going to want to do another level of baby-proofing in your home at this point. Your baby was not mobile before or was easy to scoop up while crawling, but now he is going to be on the move and getting faster. It is better to prepare now for what is about to come! Add safety gates to stairways, cover those outlets that are higher up, cover the corners of your countertops, and remove anything breakable that your baby can reach. Given time, her little hands *will find* your valuable and fragile items.

MOM TIP: Save yourself time! Download a shoe-measuring chart online from sketchers.com. Pick the shoe you're interested in, and click on it. Next, click on the size chart. A template and instructions on how to measure your child's foot to that exact shoe will appear for you to print. Then you can order the shoe online or take your child to the store, knowing her exact size. It will make your trip to the store much easier. This is also available at other online stores that sell children's shoes! Surf online to find the perfect shoes while your baby naps.

Q&A with Shanna Musick, DPT

As parents, you want to ensure that you are giving your child the best guidance, so we asked Shanna Musick, Doctor of Physical Therapy, a few questions about when your baby learns to walk. Here is what she had to say.

- *When a baby is learning to walk, should he wear socks? If so, what kind?*

  I suggest walking barefoot or in socks with grippers on the bottom. This is helpful because there is less in the way when learning to walk and he can learn to develop better balance reactions with his feet touching the ground.

- *What shoes should a toddler wear? What is best for his development?*

  After a toddler is walking, he should wear firmer, supportive shoes to give a good base of support. Robeez and other soft-soled shoes should only be worn by nonambulatory babies. (Mom translation: *Nonambulatory* means "not able to walk.")

- *What are signs that a child's feet are developing correctly? What are the signs that there is a problem?*

  The child should be walking or standing independently by 15 months. After your toddler has been walking for a few months, if his feet are overly flat or turned in, please seek out a physical-therapy evaluation from your pediatrician.

- *What is toe-walking, and how do I correct this?*

  Walking without heel contact more than 25% of the time or walking up on your toes is considered toe-walking, and this could be caused by a variety of factors, such as tight Achilles tendons (or "heel cords"), a tethered spinal cord (a rare neurological disorder caused by tissue attachments that limit the movement of the spinal cord within the spinal column),[6] sensory issues, cerebral palsy, or any combination of these.

Start by getting a referral from your pediatrician for a physical-therapy or occupational-therapy evaluation. A therapist may recommend a stretching program and/or desensitization activities or refer you to an orthopedic specialist. Some kids end up needing orthotics or surgery in extreme cases to help lengthen tight heel cords.

- *What is the most important thing you would like parents to know about healthy feet?*

I would like parents to understand the importance of good, supportive shoe wear. I recommend going to a shoe store and getting your child's shoe sized and fitted properly every time you purchase new shoes.

Baby's Sensory Systems

Baby's Ears

We conducted a survey and asked 100 parents which, if any, of their baby's sensory systems was an issue. The results showed that more than 35% of parents noticed a problem with their baby's auditory system. First, let's explore just how much your baby's auditory system is developing.

Auditory Development

Your baby is able to hear at birth—however, his hearing abilities will become more complex throughout childhood. Your baby's sound localization improves, meaning his ability to locate where a sound is coming from and if the sound is close by or far away. He's also more likely to be able to differentiate sounds in an active environment—inside a restaurant, for example, he will be able to "tune out" some noises while focusing on his parents' voices. Your baby's auditory threshold is still developing, and he will most likely respond best to your "Mommy voice" (a high-pitched voice used to give praise and affection to our babies and pets). The frequencies of higher-pitched voices make it easier for babies to distinguish individual parts of speech.

Ear Infections

Why is it that our ears are most susceptible to ear infections at the age when our auditory development is so crucially developing? Ear infections can start early—even in the womb, caused by infections in a pregnant woman. Genital herpes, toxoplasmosis, syphilis, and rubella may cause ear infections in an unborn baby. Mercury and lead, amongst many other chemicals, are known to specifically damage the developing auditory system.

Once a child is born, there are several more factors to consider. Bottle-fed babies, children exposed to second-hand smoke, and children in daycare or in multiple-child environments are more prone to ear infections, but genetics are also an underlying factor. If your baby has narrow Eustachian tubes, the chances of developing an ear infection are higher. Since ear infections are caused by bacteria or a virus, either can result in fluid buildup in the middle inner ear and through the Eustachian tube. While breastfeeding and keeping your baby home might help, there are no guarantees that your child will not get ear infections.

Signs of Ear Infection or Eustachian Tube Blockage

While not all the signs occur with every baby, look for a fever, reduced appetite, fussiness, grabbing at the ears, and possible yellow drainage. More persistent blockage may result in partial deafness. Is your child responding to her name being called? Is she babbling? Does she startle when there is a loud noise or when a siren drives by?

Ear infections are painful. If your baby has an ear infection, know that she is uncomfortable. Since ear infections are often accompanied by a sinus infection or a cold, your baby is going to need some extra tender loving care while her body fights off the infection.

What to Do?

Call your doctor immediately. It is always better to be safe than sorry. Your doctor might recommend letting your baby's body fight the infection naturally, prescribe an antibiotic, or, if the ear infections are persistent and chronic, suggest surgically inserting tubes to alleviate the frequency of the infections. Whatever the choice, it is between you and your doctor.

The good news is that there are not any conclusive studies stating that children with chronic ear infections suffer from language delays or learning disabilities in their school years. My personal experience is not consistent with their conclusions. My son had a hearing blockage (we're not sure for how long), and it has taken a very long time for him to catch up to his peers in speech, as well as in language comprehension.

Your Baby's Vestibular System

The vestibular system, which is the internal system that regulates balance and gives us a sense of spatial orientation and movement, is crucial to your baby's development at this stage. This system is what allows your baby to stand and then eventually start to walk. How do you know if your child's vestibular system is maturing on schedule? Does she sit up straight? Is she able to stand unassisted at 12 months? Is your son able to track you with his eyes while moving his head?

Your baby has most likely started doing his own vestibular stimulation, such as swaying to music while holding himself in a standing position at the coffee table, shaking his head in the car, rocking his body, or bouncing in place. Some infants enjoy a baby jumper lodged safely in a doorframe for a vestibular workout. Other children might spin their chairs at the kitchen table or crave spinning on the merry-go-round at the local park.

While some sleep experts tell parents not to rock, sway, or bounce their babies if they want them to sleep on their own, they're overlooking the significance of stimulating the baby's vestibular system, which is necessary in a baby's development. Rocking or bouncing fussy babies has been known to calm them, as well as help organize their internal systems. Activating the vestibular system can help a baby to become more alert, and it can also help decrease a baby's level of arousal. This may be why an adult instinctively sways when holding a baby. Internally, we may know to stimulate the baby's vestibular system without even being told.

You can help keep your child's vestibular system healthy as she grows. Spin her in the toddler swing at the park. Be sure to spin one way, and then, as if unwinding, spin her the other way. Always stop if your child is not enjoying the activity or if she looks like she's in discomfort. You can get a swing that is built safely for your doorway and follow all the manufacturer's instructions to ensure a safe indoor swinging experience for your child. You can hold your daughter while sitting on a teeter-totter—the up-down movement is great for getting movement going in the inner ears. Go up and down the slide with your son, or "spot him" while he does it on his own. Many activities that are fun for your child are giving his vestibular system a workout. So enjoy that time at the park or turn your home into a fun children's gym in the name of vestibular health!

Fine-Motor Skills

Your baby is most likely becoming more and more interested in lots of new things! As your baby transforms into a toddler, she will develop fine-motor skills, which are used to coordinate small movements of the fingers and hands in conjunction with the eyes. She may want to start coloring, so you can introduce finger paints—just make sure you always supervise her so she doesn't put her fingers in her mouth. If your child appears to struggle with fine-motor skills, such as pointing, turning pages in a book one at a time, or trying to grasp a crayon or marker, here are some things you can do to fine-tune those skills.

- Have her use her hands for projects and puzzles—encourage her to color and paint.
- Practice picking up small pieces of food (like cereal pieces), using her pincer grasp (thumb and index finger).
- Ask her to point to pictures in books or practice turning one page at a time in a board book.

Gross-Motor Skills

Gross-motor skills involve the use of the larger muscle groups, as well as coordination of whole-body movements. It will be helpful to give your baby opportunities to exercise, so she can develop these skills. By "exercise" I don't mean lifting weights—I'm talking about stimulating muscle movement and control with repetitive practice, which creates strength—such as jumping in a baby jumper. This will help your baby to crawl, walk, and eventually to run and jump. We're not encouraging exercise to help your baby reach milestones earlier; what we are promoting is strengthening that may help with coordination, self-esteem, and confidence when your baby does reach gross-motor milestones. The following are all good sources of gross-motor activity:

- Any sort of weight-bearing activity on her hands (crab walking, bear walking)
- Baby yoga
- Swimming with your baby can be fun for both of you, if you follow safety guidelines!
- Climbing—supervise your baby climbing up playground equipment, and help her down.

Visual-Motor Skills

Your baby's visual system will continue to develop for years to come, but it is important to stimulate the visual wiring before your baby turns 2 years old. From birth until this time, your baby's visual system is literally building itself by what your baby sees and what your baby is exposed to. This is a dance between nature and nurture that secures your baby's sight capabilities for the remainder of her life, although genetics play a role in vision, as well.[7]

Note that when you're exposing your child to pictures in books, art, and new environments, you're developing your baby's spatial perception and the ability to differentiate shapes, sizes, and colors. When you give your baby a toy or an item to play with, you are helping her develop hand-eye coordination. Through visual experimentation, your baby is stimulating visual areas of her brain that allow depth perception. If you notice your baby's eyes crossing or if she has clouding over her eyes (in the form of cataracts), please notify your pediatrician right away.

Around the age of 1 to 2 years, your child should begin looking through books on her own and enjoying being read to. She will, at times, want to page backward in the book, not always understanding how to go from beginning to end, or maybe she'll want to go back and look at something that was interesting to her. I encourage families to talk about the pictures in the books. Ask your child to point to the dog. Once she has pointed to the dog, say, "What does the dog say?" You can bark along with your child, making reading and learning fun. You may practice sign language while reading books, too. Find the flower, and then sign "flower" so your child is looking at the picture and then looking at you. She might even try to say "flower."

As your child becomes a toddler, encourage her to work puzzles. I really like Melissa & Doug puzzles, and the wooden ones with little knobs on the pieces are easier for young children to manipulate. You can point to where the puzzle piece goes, and then, if your child needs help, turn the piece for her, and help her fit it in. Eventually, she will begin to learn how to match the puzzle pieces with the pictures on the puzzle.

Other visual-motor tasks that are good to work on are stacking blocks and building simple block designs. Experiment with your child by stacking cups or big Legos and have your toddler identify the colors of the blocks. Around this age, she will begin to pick out the blue block when you ask her to!

Baby's Nose

By 1 year of age, your baby will make a face if he smells something stinky or something that he's not fond of. A fun way to develop your baby's sense of smell is to introduce new scents to him. Make sure you don't use any harmful chemicals or perfumes that can be toxic to your baby. Stick with smells of fruits and foods that would be pleasing to him and perhaps a few flowers from your front lawn. Make sure your

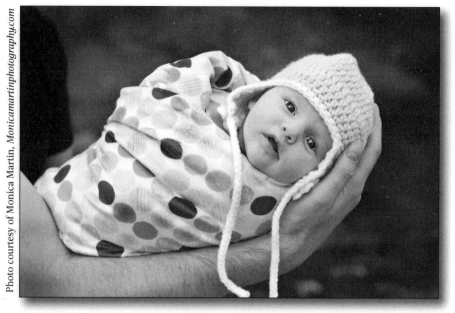

Life can be so sweet!
PAYTON SNUGGLED UP IN DADDY'S ARMS.

baby does not stick these items up his nose, either, as a trip to the emergency room is never fun if a bean gets lodged up there. Talk to your baby about smells. "This lemon smells fresh. Do you like the smell of these peppermint leaves?"

You might notice your child sniffing things, such as his toys, maybe Daddy's shoes, even his diaper. It is natural for babies to explore their world through smell. Your baby won't mind as much as you do if the smells are not pleasant. This is another way for him to differentiate items in his world. If your baby is particularly sensitive to smell, he will notice when you wash his favorite blanket, and he may get upset that the smell he was familiar with is gone. My husband pulls the blankets on our bed up over his mouth and nose at night, and I always thought that was so strange, until I read that it's the comforting scent of the blanket that helps him sleep. I now know this is something he developed as an infant and has carried through his entire life.

Baby's Taste

Around 9 months of age, your child will more than likely begin to show interest in table foods. This is because his pallet has changed, and he is able to tolerate more textured foods, like the ones we eat as adults. If your child had delays in oral-motor skills or has sensory aversions to certain textures and flavors, you may be thinking, "Heck no—my child barely eats level-one baby foods!" If your child is 1 year old and is still eating only baby foods, you need to seek out a feeding specialist to help you introduce new foods. According to Dr Kay Toomey (a world-renowned pediatric psychologist who specializes in feeding), your baby's primary source of calories during the first year of life should be breast milk or formula. That said, you should still begin to introduce rice cereal, fruits, vegetables, and meats starting around 4-6 months of age and add as you go. Your 1-year-old should now be eating small pieces of regular table food, and you can also begin to introduce cow milk, or, if your child is lactose intolerant, rice, almond, coconut, or potato milk. There are so many choices! If you're concerned about your baby's diet, as always, talk to your pediatrician and get a referral to a specialist, if needed. For more information on this topic, please read the first section in chapter 8, regarding oral aversions and picky eaters.

Baby's Tactile Sense

Remember we mentioned that your skin is your largest organ? Well, think of all the things a mobile 1-2-year-old is touching and exploring. Some children begin to get a little more defensive toward unknown things, like sticky or gooey foods, while eating. They may not want to touch the sticky cheese to pick it up or eat pudding because it's gooey. It may be best to slowly introduce your child to a variety of textures and various media (finger paints, sand, mud and dirt, and more) to help him learn to tolerate various textures on his hands and feet and in his mouth. Please make sure you ALWAYS supervise your child while playing with these media, because he is probably still sticking some things into his mouth, and you don't want him eating Play-Doh and mud (though a little dirt won't hurt!). Remember that it's okay to get messy. Not only is it good for your baby's tactile development to be covered from head to toe in spaghetti in his high chair, it also makes for an adorable photo opportunity. Now, if only there was someone else around to clean up the mess!

Baby's Proprioceptive Sense

In order to pull himself up, crawl, and walk, your child needs many of his body systems to work together at one time. One key sense is proprioception, which is the awareness of how your body is positioned and moving in space. Here is an example of how to access your proprioceptive sense. Close your eyes and reach your right arm straight out in front of you. Next, while your eyes are still closed, make your left arm do the same thing your right arm is doing. If your left arm mimics your right, then you have a good proprioceptive sense. If you are unable to make your left arm match the right, then you probably have a poor proprioceptive sense. A similar test is used by police when they test for drunk driving. They may ask a driver to close his eyes, lean his head back, and touch his nose. If his proprioceptive sense is impaired, then he won't be able to balance and find his nose with his finger, even if he's not intoxicated.

Some babies do not have a great sense of body awareness, which can cause decreased balance and coordination. That said, when learning to walk, it is typical for ALL babies to be wobbly and fall down as they learn to get their feet underneath them. They will also bump into things as they are learning to navigate around the coffee table. (This is not to be confused with a compromised sense of proprioception!)

To provide added proprioceptive input for your child, you can apply nice, deep pressure to her muscles and joints (as in a massage). You should not be hurting your child, but gentle, firm pressure on her arms, hands, legs, and feet can feel good. You can pretend you're making a sandwich on her. Start by pretending to rub mustard on her back in smooth strokes. Then "chop up" some tomatoes with soft chopping motions, and place them on her back. (Make sure to stop if your child doesn't enjoy this.) You can use the tips of your fingers to "sprinkle " salt and pepper. Make sure you use deep pressure, because light touch can be disorienting to some children—even painful.

Your child will naturally get proprioceptive input by doing things like crawling, walking, jumping, sitting down, crunching and chewing foods, pushing toys around, and getting great-big hugs from you! She will also get proprioceptive input by lounging in a beanbag chair or a net swing.

Sleep Cycles Change

As your baby gets older, his sleep cycles will change, and he will begin to sleep through the night, or at least for a longer duration during the night. You've most likely read or heard about the "fussy hour" that seems to posses your baby around dinnertime. "Fussy o'clock" can strike just as your husband or partner is getting home from work or as you are arriving home, and it is not fun for any of you. This can be particularly tough if one of you wants to interact with the baby and you are stimulating him, while your baby is showing signs of needing to go to bed. Try to be mindful that your baby's sleep schedule has to take precedence over your own. There will be years and years for Dad to bond with the child. Maybe he can get up early to feed the baby before work, and you can catch some extra sleep! As your baby enters toddlerhood, he should start transitioning from two naps a day to one. Every child is different, and as a parent, you will determine when your child is ready for this.

Baby Self-Soothing

If your baby has established a sleep cycle and then, all of a sudden, he starts waking up again in the night, this could be due to teething or is just part of his growth. If your baby uses a pacifier, help guide his hands to it and allow him to put it into his mouth to help soothe him back to sleep. This can help with teething pain, as well.

Your baby is constantly growing and learning new skills, so it may be hard for him to sleep when he has just discovered he can move his hand.

Every little new thing can be exciting for a baby and disrupt sleep cycles. Your baby is just that—a baby! It may take time for him to learn to soothe himself. Keep at it, Mom and Dad—he will learn with your help.

The Security Blanket

The security blanket or "lovey" of choice is often something that the parents love as much as the child. It may be a blanket from a favorite aunt or a stuffed animal from a favorite story. As parents, it makes us feel good to see our child attached to something we have fond memories of. The lovey provides security for your baby and addresses many other sensory needs. Is the lovey soft, and does your baby rub it to feel its texture while soothing herself to sleep? Does your child keep the lovey snuggled up next to her tightly for that proprioceptive feedback? You may find that your child will sniff her lovey or security blanket as she is soothing herself into sleep mode.

Your child might not gravitate to the lovey of your choice, and you're going to have to allow her to select her own source of comfort. The lovey can be there when you cannot. And she may grow out of one lovey or transition to another item of choice. What I like best about the security blanket is that it doesn't seem to generate quite as much controversy as other items when it comes to letting your child keep it as she grows into adolescence. If the child is allowed to keep this item as long as she needs it, she will often stash it in a drawer or her closet once she outgrows it (but it's always there).

Where Is Your Baby Sleeping?

Some babies naturally sleep well anywhere, anytime, any place. This may not be true for you and your baby. Many parents have their infants sleep in bed with them or in a crib in their room. We support whatever works for you. As your baby is now getting older, he should be able to sleep alone in his crib and maybe even his own room. Some cultures and parents encourage "co-sleeping," where the child sleeps with the parents or even a sibling. These adjustment periods can be tough on both you and your baby. Make sure you plan for these transitions, and do not be hard on yourself if there are regressions. Some baby-sleep experts make it seem as if your baby will never learn to sleep through the night or transition into a crib if she sleeps in the bed with you at first, but babies and children are resilient and they do adapt (some more easily than others). Try not to be hard on yourself, you're learning too!

Do you rely on the swing for your baby's naptime, or does she fall asleep in the car? While this is okay sometimes, sleep experts agree that a baby gets the best sleep in her own bed. You need to make sure she gets deep sleep and not just a catnap or a light rest.

Your Sleep

At times, you will feel like you are constantly on Sleep Watch, always checking for signs that your baby is tired and then adjusting to his sleep cycles as they change. Whether your baby is sleeping in a crib or with you in bed, why don't you nap while your baby naps, too? Many moms try to get a bunch of stuff done during naptime, but we suggest using at least one of those naps to get your own shut-eye. You also need to get enough sleep. You may be excited to finally find yourself getting almost 7 hours of sleep a night! Yay! Make sure you are continuing to take care of yourself, so that you have the energy to keep up with your growing baby.

Play

Play is a child's primary occupation. This interaction and stimulation gives the child the opportunity to develop skills that are the foundation for future skill building, such as problem-solving skills, manipulation of objects, and increasing attention to task. A child must be intrinsically motivated to play, but, as a parent, you can set up situations where you provide opportunities for appropriate play interactions to occur. At this age, your child will not understand symbolic play, which is where one object is "substituted" for another—such as using a banana as a telephone. He has not learned what items are and what they're used for. Right now, he's an explorer!

Social Play

Now that your child is 1 year old, he is beginning to interact with other children in different ways. He learns from watching others, and this can help him grow developmentally. If your child has cousins, neighbors, or friends at daycare, have him play with them often. The kids can be older than your child or even younger.

Children around 1-2 years of age get very protective of their toys and don't want share. Or, maybe they only want the toy that someone else is playing with. They're too young to completely understand the concept of sharing, but these are great teaching opportunities for you to start showing that if they do share, they get the toy back. Try to turn sharing into a game.

Developmentally Appropriate Toys: 1 to 2 Years

* *Coloring with crayons.* As a therapist, I suggest crayons and not markers, because the child gets more pressure and feedback from coloring with a crayon on paper.

OCCUPATIONAL THERAPIST TIP: I will sometimes break the crayons so that one piece is about three-fourths of the crayon length, and I save the other quarter for when the child gets a little stronger with her fine-motor skills. This way, the child is encouraged to hold the crayon closer to the tip, instead of holding it way back at the end of the crayon. Also, when picking out markers, I like the Pip-Squeaks markers because they are one-half the size of a regular marker.

- *Books!* You can't read enough books to your child.

- *Puzzles of all kinds*—especially wooden puzzles with knobs that the child can manipulate. There are puzzles that make fun noises and ones that are textured. Puzzles with locks are complex for your baby to master, and they stimulate different problem-solving skills.

- *Balls for throwing and learning to catch.* You can start by rolling a ball back and forth on the ground between the two of you.

- *Beanbags for tossing into a bucket or laundry basket.* Your baby may be more interested in holding them and feeling them right now, but as she gets older, she can work on her visual-perception skills and aim. This also assists in the development of depth perception and spatial awareness. These are big skills for your little one to learn.

- *Blow bubbles for your toddler to try and pop.* She can reach out and point to them with her finger. I've never met a child who doesn't love bubbles. Reaching for them with a finger assists in the development of fine-motor skills, visual spatial awareness, and impulse control.

- *Bath toys*—try letters for the walls, bath crayons, or paints.

- *Baths.* Baths are great for your child's proprioceptive sense, as he's getting constant feedback from the water, telling him where his body is in space. Kicking and splashing gives his muscles a workout, while alphabet sponges help him learn about letters. The water temperature stimulates the tactile sense and the child's internal regulation system. If there are bubbles and scents, his olfactory system is activated, as well as his vision. Think of all the sensory input he's processing at once! Who knew the bath was such a grand sensory classroom?

- *Riding toys.* These toys, such as a bike that you push with your feet, activate your child's core muscles (as he sits up) and his legs (as he pushes off the ground to move forward). He's having to steer, too, and learn about running into the couch. All these lessons will come in handy when he's getting his driver's license, years from now. I like Disney's Cars McQueen Ride-On Toy, available at target.

- *Cars, trains, and planes.* Push the cars along the ground. Swing the planes in the air. Make horn noises and wind swooshes. Build train tracks for your child's train.

- *Tents and playhouses.* Oh what fun to go in and out of a tent 100 times!

- *Stacking blocks and/or large Lego blocks.* Cardboard blocks are a dream for little ones to stack. Pretend you are the "Three Little Pigs" and build a house. Then, the wolf can come and knock it down. Build it again and again and again.

- *Get outside and take adventure walks!* What colors are the flowers? How big is the ocean? Do your neighbors have a barking dog? Even sidewalk cracks are interesting at this age. You never know what kind of bug will crawl out.

Developmental Milestones, 1 to 2 Years

12-14 MONTHS

Gross- and Fine-Motor Development
- Sits first when she falls
- May begin walking alone (Every child begins walking at different times. If your child isn't walking by 15 or 16 months, then you may want to seek out a professional—your pediatrician may recommend consultation with a physical therapist.)
- Bangs two objects together
- Begins marking on paper with crayons
- Puts three or more blocks into a container
- Can pick up a ball and release it (maybe even toss it)

Visual-Motor Development
- Helps put on clothing by holding out her arms and helps take off her clothing
- Imitates scribbling when demonstrated for her
- Stacks two blocks

Speech and Language Development
- Points to a few body parts
- Says more words every month
- Answers "yes or no" questions by nodding her head

Social and Cognitive Development
- Is more than likely impulsive
- Is unable to control all her body movements (she may be clumsy and fall a lot)
- Is easily distracted
- Imitates simple things she sees adults do
- Looks for adults to watch and be proud of something she does
- Will take turns throwing a small ball back and forth

- Will show a preference for a particular toy or activity
- Finds an object when you hide it under something
- May throw tantrums more frequently
- Needs and expects routines
- Can bring a spoon to her mouth when it has food on it
- Holds a cup with handles

15-16 MONTHS

Gross- and Fine-Motor Development
- Walks with more stability
- Begins fast walking
- Crawls up stairs, still goes backwards down stairs
- Walks sideways
- Throws a ball forward
- Bends down to a squat and then stands back up
- Walks up stairs holding onto a rail with both feet on the step
- Places round pegs into holes
- Scribbles and paints
- Points with an index finger
- Puts small objects in a container, like Cheerios into a cup

Speech and Language Development
- Points to objects and pictures
- Says two to three words
- Listens to simple stories
- Follows simple directions

Social and Cognitive Development
- Gives a toy to an adult for help or for interaction
- Begins to show a sense of humor
- Enjoys being the center of attention
- Gives hugs and kisses to family members
- Becomes very independent—enters the "no" stage

- May indicate discomfort over a soiled diaper
- Sleeps 10-12 hours a night and has one nap a day
- Takes off her hat and socks and helps more with taking off her shirt
- Begins to scoop food with a spoon and bring it to her mouth
- Is unable to share toys with other children at times

17-18 MONTHS

Gross- and Fine-Motor Development
- Walks backwards
- Walks downstairs holding onto a rail, with both feet on the step
- Stands on one foot with help
- Picks up a toy off the floor without falling
- Pulls a toy behind her as she walks
- Climbs into a chair, turns, and sits
- Walks and carries an object
- Explores with her hands more frequently than with her mouth
- Uses a pincer grasp (thumb and index finger) consistently to pick up small objects
- Uses two hands on objects
- Puts pegs into a pegboard

Visual Development
- Points at distant objects
- Tracks moving objects (like a ball coming toward her)
- Tries to kick a ball
- Throws a small ball approximately 3 feet while standing still

Speech and Language Development
- Speaks six to 20 or more recognizable words (or uses sign language if speech is delayed)
- Enjoys nursery rhymes
- Babbles to herself while playing
- Knows three to four body parts

Social and Cognitive Development

- Drinks from an open cup with a little liquid in it without spilling
- Puts a hat on
- May refuse foods she previously liked (especially when teething)
- Removes shoes
- Alternates between independence and dependence on a caregiver
- Likes to do things on her own, but likes to have an adult nearby
- Imitates familiar actions, like sweeping, reading a book, and vacuuming

19-21 MONTHS

Gross- and Fine-Motor Development

- Kicks a ball forward
- Pushes and pulls objects
- Walks down stairs holding a railing or a parent's hand
- Creeps backwards down stairs
- Can carry toys when walking
- Builds a block tower of four blocks
- Scribbles on paper
- Strings a bead

Visual Development

- Scoops food from one container to another
- Feeds herself with a spoon and fork without spilling too much

Language Development

- Echoes the last word spoken to her
- Talks/babbles to herself while playing
- Starts to combine words, like "more milk"
- Makes animal sounds
- Understands simple verbs (ie, eat, sleep)

Social and Cognitive Development

- Raises and holds a cup with two hands
- Unzips and can sometimes zip a large zipper
- Can tell the difference between edible and inedible objects
- Begins to give up the bottle sometime before 24 months

22-24 MONTHS

Gross- and Fine-Motor Development

- Walks with legs together
- Stands on tiptoes
- Jumps with two feet in place
- Throws a small ball
- Builds a six-block tower
- Imitates vertical strokes
- Imitates circular strokes
- Strings three beads together
- Turns pages in a book one at a time
- Picks up tiny objects, such as crumbs
- Removes a wrapper from food before eating it (ie, a cupcake)

Visual Development

- Kicks a ball forward with either foot without support
- Names familiar toys from a 10-foot distance
- Points at things in a book on command

Language Development

- Engages in pretend play
- Asks "What's that?" questions
- Sings nursery rhymes and songs
- Uses 50 or more recognizable words, understands more than 300 words
- Puts together two or more words to formulate sentences
- Refers to herself by her own name

- Points and says body parts
- Understands simple commands and conversation

Social and Cognitive Development

- Plays with food
- Chews food completely
- Clings to caregiver when tired or afraid
- Demands a lot of caregiver's attention
- Delays sleeping by demanding things
- Washes and dries hands with a little help
- Has particular food preferences
- Throws tantrums when frustrated
- Is possessive about toys, has a hard time sharing

Developmental Concerns

If you have been noticing that your child has not been meeting his motor milestones and you are feeling concerned, definitely talk to your pediatrician about it. If your child seems to be a few months behind in a lot of different areas (gross-motor, fine-motor, and social/emotional skills) or is really delayed in motor skills, then ask your pediatrician to refer you for a physical-therapy, occupational-therapy, or speech-therapy evaluation, depending on what is going on with your child. Even if you have your child evaluated and you are told that nothing is wrong, it is better than waiting too long when your child is struggling with meeting his developmental milestones.

Don't panic! It's all going to be okay, and if you don't agree with what your pediatrician has said, then get a second opinion. As a therapist, I see children who may be a little behind and they don't need therapy, but I give parents a home program to work on and have them come back in 6 months if things are still looking delayed. Other times, I will see a toddler who is obviously delayed in motor skills and has sensory-processing issues or behavioral issues, and the mom or dad says that the pediatrician kept telling them their baby was fine and they shouldn't worry. All the research says that early intervention is best if there is any chance your child may struggle with a delay, so speak up for your child and get him evaluated if you are feeling concerned. It's better to be safe than sorry!

CHAPTER FIVE

Baby's Caregivers

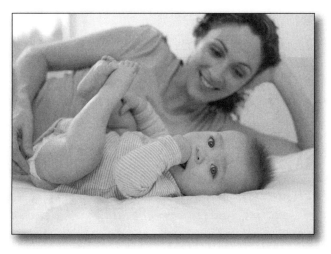

Everything our babies do is amazing,
we could watch them all day!

CAIUS AND NAOMI

Babysitters, Nannies, and Daycare

EVERY NOW AND THEN, YOU'RE GOING TO HAVE TO LEAVE YOUR MOST
valuable possession and go to work, go to the doctor, have coffee with
girlfriends, or take a spin class. Some parents find it extremely hard to

leave their baby, and they cope with separation-anxiety issues. This is entirely understandable and natural, as we all have the need to protect our babies. It can be scary to trust your baby in the arms of someone else, especially someone new. Other moms live for time away from their baby and will leave their child with the plumber if he agrees to strap the baby monitor to his tool belt. It's different strokes for different folks. As all babies are different, we have come to realize that all parents are different, too.

Babysitters

Babysitters used to be strictly old ladies and high-school girls. Now they are everything in between, including other mothers, teachers, and nurses. Some are looking for additional income, and others make a career out of taking care of children. It is up to you as the parent to decide what works best for your family. Do you have high-school girls on your block that you're comfortable with? If so, have them come play with your baby while you're at home doing chores or getting ready and see how they interact with the baby. Observe how they talk to him, hold him, and play with him. Are they comfortable or awkward with your baby? Start with quick outings to ensure that both the baby and the young babysitter are okay with one another and that the babysitter will call for help if needed. Also, set guidelines that there are to be no boyfriends, no texting, and no Facebook while you're gone, unless the baby is sleeping. An advantage is that babies are usually interested in older kids and enjoy attention from teenagers.

A popular substitute is sharing babysitting duties with other mothers. This is a way to keep costs down by bartering babysitting services with the added benefit that your child is being socialized at the same time. Make sure that you and the other moms you're dividing time with are fair about duties and expectations. You don't want a mom watching your baby for an hour and then dropping off her five kids for a weekend. Keep track of the amount of hours you're sharing so that one of you doesn't end up getting burnt out and resentful. Keep your baby's sensory needs in mind, as well. You don't want to drop him into a sensory disaster if he's not used to a house of chaos. If your baby prefers a calm environment with maybe only one other child, don't leave him with the mom who has four boys and a house full of dogs and ferrets. Also make sure you're not leaning on a mom who already has her hands full but thinks she's able to take on one more child. You want to make sure your baby is going to get proper attention and not be left with a 5-year-old to watch him. Also, know if this mom is going to be taking your baby on errands with her and her children. If you're leaving your baby with her, find out what is on her agenda for the day, as well.

If your child has special needs or you're concerned about leaving him without a trained professional, there are many teachers, tutors, caregivers, and nurses that offer babysitting services. You can find these women through an agency, which we recommend because they can do background checks and screening for you. We also recommend talking to their references. It never hurts to be too careful, and if she's legitimate, she won't mind having you check up on her. We find that most babysitters truly love children, and many have a gift of nurturing and bringing out the best in our little ones. You can find women who used to be nannies for a particular family, and that family has grown up, and you will find women who grew up with their parents running a daycare, so they know how to get down and have fun with your little one.

Nanny

If only we could purchase a Mary Poppins at the online Disney store and have her delivered to our homes with her rosy cheeks and cheery disposition, or perhaps a Maria from "The Sound of Music" to arrive and teach our children to sing in clothes she sewed from our old curtains. Life would be incredibly easy. But, in reality, the task of hiring a nanny is far more complex. You want to find an au pair who has the same mindset as you and who will be consistent with your routine.

As a family, make a list of priorities of important qualities you want in your nanny. Also make a list of rules and guidelines that you and Nanny are going to follow. Here are some examples.

- *Priority List, Example 1:*

  Nanny will be kind, have a college degree in childhood development, and be able to work every other weekend.

- *Priority List, Example 2:*

  Nanny will speak Spanish to our child, have children of her own, and have a driver's license.

See what I mean? You can pick the priorities that apply to your family. After that, you will want a list of rules and guidelines that you and the Nanny will follow.

- *Example Rules and Guidelines List:*

  When Mommy gets home from work, Nanny will stay 15 minutes for transition time and tell Mommy important information from the day. When Mommy has to work late, Nanny will get $20 overtime pay for every hour that she stays past 6 pm. Mommy will call Nanny and ask if this overtime is okay on that day but will make an effort to schedule overtime hours in advance.

You may be wondering how any of this is sensory related. It's to do with organization. It's hard for a child to regulate his sensory system and nervous system if there are not established boundaries and routines. If the child is worried that Mommy isn't coming home and his Nanny is pacing by the door as she waits to leave for her dinner date, then your child will be unsettled and upset. If the Nanny doesn't know what is expected of her and she darts out the door as Mommy enters, then the child doesn't have time to adjust. Without getting too scientific about it, your child's central nervous system works together with the peripheral nervous system to play a fundamental role in the control of behavior. So, your behavior and your Nanny's behavior affects your child's internal systems and his ability to control his behavior. It's food for thought.

Sensory Nanny Checklist

Here are some things to consider as a parent and president of managing your child's senses and environments:

- *Ears*

  Does your nanny speak the same language as you do? Is she fluent? While it may be a good idea to teach your child another language from birth, if your child has an auditory issue, this is going to further disrupt his development of sound and language.

  Does your nanny have a nasal voice or a screechy voice that is uncomfortable to your baby's ears? Or, does your nanny speak softly, and your child can't hear her easily?

- *Nose*

  Does the nanny smell like musk perfume? Or, does she smoke in her car and cover it up with a spray? If your child has a sensitive nose, stop and consider whether Nanny has a smelly coat that she wears every day. Uncomfortable smells can be overwhelming for your child and even cause headaches.

- *Taste*

  Since the nanny will be providing meals for your child throughout the day, will she meet the nutritional needs of your child in tasty ways that your child will want to eat, without it being a daily torture?

- *Touch*

  Will the nanny encourage your baby or child to feel new media, such as paint, glue, feathers, and sand? Will she use a trip to the grocery store to show your baby the different textures of fruits and vegetables?

  Will the nanny work on helping your child to dress, including practicing the fine-motor tasks involved with buttons, zippers, snaps, and fasteners?

- *Proprioception*

  Hugs and comfort are important. Is the nanny comfortable showing love and affection to your child throughout the day? Will she snuggle on the couch while watching TV? Will she give a few squeezes before sending him off to play on the jungle gym at the park? Will she hold his hand while they're crossing the street? Will she hold him if he falls down and scrapes his knee?

- *Milestones*

  Will the nanny observe and participate in helping your baby reach milestones? Will she allot an appropriate amount of tummy time? Will the nanny place toys on the floor in front of your baby and encourage him to crawl?

If you expect your nanny to care for your child or children 24/7, clean your house, and make your meals in exchange for room and board, you're creating an unbalanced relationship in your home and setting an unwelcome example for your child. In our opinion, it's not healthy for your family to expect so much of a nanny. Your nanny should be hired as your nanny, period. His or her only focus is to care for your child or children, and you must set boundaries as to the hours that the nanny will be working. As you know, caring for children is the hardest job in the universe and requires endless energy, compassion, and tenacity. You do not want your children to become attached to your nanny, only to have her get burned out because you ask her to stay late every night of the week so you and your husband can go to dinner.

Have a contract and a set of rules for both parties to reference. If you ask your nanny to stay late or work on a weekend, then have an overtime-pay schedule set up in advance so your nanny doesn't grow to resent you. That said, your nanny is your employee—not your best friend—and not your punching bag. Keep it professional and maintain a working relationship with an open door of communication about the child or children.

Now, how does the nanny fit into your child's sensory world? Well, if she is spending most of the day with your baby or child, then she needs to be aware of his sensory needs. The nanny will be able to tell you if your child won't eat certain textures, if your child puts his head on the ground to look at toys, if your child has tantrums when switching activities, or if he refuses to wear gloves when it's cold outside. The nanny can also tell you how the child acts during the day when he's out with people other than immediate family members. Does your nanny meet up with other nannies and children at the park? Does your child engage with other children? Does your child share with other children? Is he genuinely interested in playing with his peers or does he stare off into the trees and focus on a leaf for an hour? Is your child speaking at the same level as the other children at the park? Does your child avoid exploring on the slide and swings and prefer to stay on the ground or in the sandbox? Is your child bothered by the noise level of the other children? Does your child freak out every time the nanny puts fruit in the blender for his afternoon snack?

Make your nanny your copilot in your child's sensory experience. Encourage her to be observant of your child's idiosyncrasies. Your nanny may catch a problem before you do, and she may be able to evaluate your child from a more objective (and less emotional) perspective.

Like your baby, the nanny is going to want to fill her days with activities so she doesn't go stir crazy. Make sure you provide learning experiences for her to do with your baby. If she has ideas or suggestions for learning tools to use with your baby, be open to her taking an interest in your child's development. Please see our chapters on appropriate toys and learning tools for suggestions on items for your home.

Teach the nanny to be consistent with your rules and boundaries in the home. During your trial period with her, have her observe a day in the life in your home so she can see the structure and way you run your household. Do you use a visual schedule with your child? Teach the nanny how to use it.

Nanny Cam

Odds are that it is not legal in your state to keep your nanny under surveillance without her consent, and any recordings may not be used in a court of law against your nanny. That said, with technology at your fingertips (my 8-year-old has an iPod Nano with a camera), more and more families are using video as a way to help children and to show parents what is going on when they can't be there. No longer are video cameras only for plays and dance recitals, when Dad can't get away from the office.

One nanny I'm friends with uses the camera with the child she watches, often for the child's team of specialists that are monitoring and tracking his progress, as well as for teaching others. Another friend of mine has a nanny cam in her baby's nursery that the nanny is aware of, and she knows the mom enjoys being able to see her baby during the day. The nanny is fine with it and will wave to the mom and hold the baby up before putting him down for his nap. There is not a trust issue, it's purely the mother loving her child and wanting to see him.

Some children are now enjoying the program Skype on their computers to communicate with their parents at work with the help of the nanny. See *www.skype.com* for more details. It can be comforting for children to have their parents available to them during the day, even if it's during lunchtime or when the parent is able to take a break from work.

Daycare

Picking a daycare is serious business and is something that you have hopefully been researching for months before selecting an option. There are endless things to consider, including location, prices, child-to-provider ratio, staff turnover rate, home setting or institutional daycare facility, and safety and emergency procedures. However, we are going to focus on the sensory aspects of your daycare choice when you are evaluating your options.

Try to find a daycare that is consistent to your lifestyle. The one in your neighborhood or the one provided at your workplace might not be the right fit for you and your baby. Are you flexible and spontaneous? You may need a daycare that allows parent visits at unpredictable hours. Do you have a set work schedule from 6 am to 6 pm? You will most likely want a daycare with extended hours and a set staff that you and your baby can build a relationship with.

Spend some time with the staff members, and observe them in action before you make your choice. You'll want the people looking after your baby to be people you would want to spend your day with. All day.

Inside Daycare

How does it smell in there? Is it fresh and clean, or do you smell cleaning products or mildew? Is there a hint of dirty diaper smell lingering or synthetic sprays masking odors? Is it bright and cheerful? Is there natural light shining in the windows? Are there interesting and educational decorations (but not too many)? How often are decorations changed to provide new stimulation and learning opportunities?

Is it organized and clutter free? Daycare kids are usually taught to put items away after use, a skill that is useful throughout life.

Where is feeding time conducted? Will your baby learn table skills as she grows up?

Is this a daycare for your baby, but not for when she turns two? Will you want to move her into a new environment in a few years to meet her growing needs?

Is it noisy in there? Are there scheduled quiet times? Will your baby have a quiet area in which to sleep? Will the daycare turn on some white noise for your baby if that's what she needs to be able to sleep? Is there a quiet area if your baby or toddler needs some time to regroup and regulate? Is there someplace with a beanbag where she can rest and look at a book?

Is there a large rug for her to have tummy time on and explore? Are there places for your baby to pull herself up? Are there cars and trains for her to push? Are there blocks to stack and build? Do they have toys where your child can fit shapes through holes? Do they have puzzles and a variety of books?

Is there a variety of sensory toys for your baby to play with to develop her tactile sense? Are there different fabrics, textures, shapes, and consistencies? How often are new and different toys brought into the mix? Does the facility trade toys with other daycares to keep the children stimulated and learning new things?

Is there a ball pit? Are there playhouses or tents?

Are there ample pretend-play costumes and accessories? Is there a pretend kitchen? Pretend construction tools? Is there an area for puppet shows and small performances?

How much TV and video time do they allow at the daycare? What hands-on games will they be playing with your baby? Do they have music time?

It's a lot to think about, but try and look around your baby's daycare with a child's eyes and senses and make sure that there is plenty to do and that he will stay on target with his sensory and developmental milestones.

Outside Daycare

Is the daycare on a busy street? Does the noise from neighbors carry over to the daycare? Is there a grassy area for your baby to explore? Ask about pesticides and chemicals used on the lawn and trees. Is there a nontoxic sand box with shovels and sifters? Is there a cement area for your baby to learn to ride a tricycle and play hopscotch as she gets older?

Playhouses provide hours of entertainment for little ones. Does this daycare have one outdoors? Do they have a sand and water station? These are great for developing your baby's tactile sense.

Do they have scooters for your baby to scoot on or to push a doll in to work on her motor skills?

Is there shade from trees or an awning?

Do they have themes where they work on certain activities for times of the year? During warmer times, do they allow water play outside and can everyone bring their bathing suits? In the colder months, do the kids bundle up and still get some outside time? (Not if it's freezing cold or raining, but it's still nice to have some fresh air as long as your baby is dressed appropriately.)

Swings are a great outdoor activity, and baby swings support little ones as they get some linear vestibular input. Most children really enjoy swinging. Make sure any outside equipment is in tip-top shape and not falling apart or rusting.

Siblings and Other Family Members

There are unlimited combinations of what makes a family, so we're going to look at big families, small families, and individual family members (even the ones you don't like!) from a sensory perspective.

Sensory Disasters

A charming gentleman told me how growing up in a big family was a wonderful experience, but it was a sensory disaster. A house full of kids can be a great experience for countless reasons. We love big, happy homes, and we're here to provide suggestions on how to keep your home sensory friendly and avoid sensory disasters.

You may have one child who craves football and wrestling with Dad, and then you have another child who gravitates towards books and pottery. You will find yourself with a frustrated child if you try to force him to be on the soccer team when all he wants is a paintbrush and an art class. How do you balance between heavy-metal concerts and garden retreats if you have both types of sensory systems under one roof? If you watched the now-cancelled show "Jon and Kate Plus 8," you're familiar with Kate's practice of spending quality time with each child. We know it can be hard to find quality time, *period,* let alone divided evenly amongst family members. One suggestion would be to take turns with events and outings that the family does together. Take a trip to a theme park for your sensory-seeking kids, and then make the next outing an Indian reservation tour and nature hike for your sensory-sensitive ones. Work on all your children's sensory systems. If your partner is a thrill seeker, have him take the kids that enjoy water parks out for a day of fun, and you take the kids who enjoy less sensory stimulation to a local children's discovery center.

It doesn't take a big family to have a sensory disaster. If your home is hectic, unorganized, and loud, regardless of size, it's not the sensory sanctuary some kids crave. No one is suggesting that you walk on eggshells in your own home, just take notice if your child isn't sleeping all night because of a sibling's rock music. If your child shies away from activities you have planned and requests to stay home in her room, recognize that the activities may serve as sensory overload for your child.

Sensory Nightmares

Do you have a family member who is really hard on your child's sensory system? It can be stressful if your Aunt Hilda is always squeezing your sensory-sensitive toddler. Do you have an uncle that drinks and slurs angrily at family get-togethers? Or is there a family member who is cold and judgmental when your child is just being a typical, curious toddler? While there is no way around having to deal with these types of people when you are in a group environment, such as a holiday get-together, a religious event, or a family reunion, you should protect your child's interest over that of your grouchy step-grandpa, who always wants to toss your baby in the air. If you're not comfortable, just say that she's not feeling well, and whisk her to another area of the party.

MOM TIP: It's not always easy to avoid these sensory vampires, but we do encourage you to keep your distance when you can. You don't always have to subject yourself or your children to toxic people just because they are family, extended family, or even friends.

Sensory Refuge

Whether your family is big or small, all of you need to have a sensory refuge. Perhaps you can have a room in the house that is calming and quiet and is an area for family members to recollect themselves. Everyone needs space to think and just "be." Can you reserve a bedroom where your child can safely and quietly look at a book or color? If you don't have a place in your home that is reserved for a peaceful retreat, then maybe you can designate an area outside in your yard, underneath a large oak tree.

Pets

You may have had your animals for a number of years before having a baby, and, as you've found out, having animals and kids together can be an adjustment. We have learned that a lot of things you may have been oblivious to before will grate on your nerves and senses. Here are some tips on helping "Fido" and your baby's world merge and some things to factor in if you're considering adding to your urban farm.

Two things are a guarantee: Your animal will eat, and your animal will poop. In any local pet store, you can seek out a food that is tasty for your pet, while the smell of it won't make you nauseous. There are foods to help your pet's digestion, for a reduction in poop production—but there will always be poop: regular stools and diarrhea, and perhaps even vomiting. Most likely, the one staying home with baby is the one who gets to clean this mess up, so invest in some gloves and plastic bags. That Diaper Champ can be used for animal poop, too! I've found that putting baking powder into the bottom of your trash can help keep odors under control, as well. You will have to dump your trash daily if there is any poop in it. Do not let this sit in your kitchen or laundry room overnight, emitting toxins into the air in your home.

We recommend cleaning up all indoor animal-related accidents with nontoxic cleaning products. This way, you protect your senses and your animal's senses, as well as your baby's senses. (See chapter 9 for more information on toxins in the home.) Remember that even if your baby isn't mobile yet, she will be soon. She'll be crawling and then walking exactly where your animal had an accident. It's imperative that you clean it up quickly, completely, and as safely as possible.

Birds

Beautiful birds with their pretty, colorful feathers are usually pretty noisy. They squawk, tweet, and chirp, and some even talk. They can rattle their cages and enjoy a whistle or bell from time to time. Birds are not for the auditory sensitive.

Cats

Felines are known for their independence, which can make for a great pet if you're gone at work all day. The cons are that they are also known for their dander, stinky cat box, fur balls, clawing, and scratching. Good news ladies, you get to pass over cat-box cleaning duties while pregnant and nursing to keep you and your baby safe from the risk of acquiring toxoplasmosis (a parasitic infection that can be transmitted through contact with a cat's fecal matter). Many children are allergic to cat dander, so watch your baby for signs of a runny nose, irritated eyes, or dark circles under the eyes. These mostly nocturnal animals may also keep your family awake if they're constantly playing throughout the night. You need your sleep, and so does your baby. Maybe kitty can sleep in the garage. Smelly litter boxes are not recommended for the olfactory (nose) sensitive. The litter box can be moved to the garage, and you'll have to make sure you clean it out frequently to decrease the smell. The trade-off is that the soft tactile input and companionship you'll get in return is very rewarding for both kids and adults, as is the bond your child will form with your pet.

OCCUPATIONAL THERAPIST TIP: Animals are so good for kids, especially for those with sensory difficulties. They read people's cues and can sense when a baby or young child is in distress. I have seen both dogs and cats help calm people down when they were upset.

Dogs

Oh how we love our dogs! This favorite pet is often forgiven for its dander, the hair it sheds everywhere, its incessant barking, and its rambunctious and playful demeanor because of its unwavering loyalty and love. Dogs dote on their owners, and how can you not love that? However, dogs aren't for everyone, and they can be a sensory challenge. Their dander can be potent and tough on a family member with allergies. They're often unaware of their size and can knock over your baby while she's learning to walk. Parents are oddly oblivious to the strong jaws and teeth of their dogs, thinking that their cute and cuddly companion wouldn't hurt anyone.

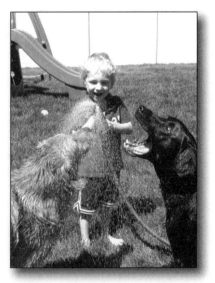

What could be more exciting for a little boy than a dog and a hose?

EVAN, 3 YEARS OLD

Once the dog encounters a toddler holding a ham sandwich, however, all bets are off. Some dogs can become jealous of a new baby, and others are oblivious to anything other than their food bowl. There are many resources to help you with your dog if you're having behavioral problems while you introduce a baby into the mix. We suggest getting these under control as quickly as possible so that your baby and dog(s) may have a healthy and solid relationship as they grow up.

A common mistake that people make is bringing home a guard dog for their family and then expecting the stay-at-home mom to walk the dog and the baby in the stroller. This can be a disaster if Mom cannot handle the dog and if the dog is extremely territorial and protective of the baby. Be sure to research the different breeds to find a suitable dog for you and your family. You can always get a terrier and invest in an alarm system.

If you're thinking of buying a cute little miniature dog to put sweaters on, be sure to research how yappy your little prince could be. Keep all of your family members' auditory sensitivities in mind before purchasing a 24-hour barking toy. There's usually a pretty strict no-return policy.

Service dogs can be extremely helpful for those who have sensory issues. They're most commonly used with the blind. They're amazing for veterans returning from war who need help with traumatic flashbacks and disorientation, and they're now commonly used to aid children with autism. Look into your local service-dog agencies if you think that having one of these dogs would be helpful to your family. Or, see if they've got any dogs that didn't pass their rigorous tests! They'll be highly trained, and maybe they just can't see as well or they have one shorter leg. There is a difference between service dog, therapy dog/pet, and companion dog/pet. Make sure you address your family's needs if you are acquiring one of these types of animals.

Ferret

Ferrets can sometimes run free in a house and are treated somewhat like cats and dogs. Just follow sanitary guidelines on cleaning up after your ferret(s), and, as a precautionary measure, keep it out of your baby's or toddler's room. You will have to train your ferret to use the litter box and do what is called "nip-training," so your ferret doesn't take a bite out of the baby.

Fish

A word to the wise—goldfish die, sometimes before you even get them home. As someone who has had a "magic" spotted goldfish for 5 years (who periodically makes a trip to the pet store for a cleaning), do not bring home a fish in "The Little Mermaid" aquarium unless you're ready to talk to your little one about life and death (a concept they won't easily grasp at this early stage). If it's a pet your child keeps in her bedroom, she may be more attached to it than if you have a family aquarium in the living room because it's Daddy's hobby. If you're going more for the family aquarium, with either salt water or fresh water—fantastic.

OCCUPATIONAL THERAPIST TIP: Fish are known to be mesmerizing and soothing. Hospitals and doctors' and dentists' offices use fish tanks to help soothe their patients in the waiting room. This can be very helpful for a kid with overwhelming sensory issues, who may have difficulty self-soothing.

After watching "Finding Nemo," your child will be even more thrilled about having a fish for a pet. Just make sure your baby doesn't bang on the glass with her hand or a toy, in case the glass breaks or falls on her. Always take precautionary safety measures.

Know that fish can be a lot of work. You have to clean their tanks often, and maintaining the proper amount of algae can be a science experiment in itself. If you don't like getting your hands wet, this isn't the pet for you.

Gerbils, Hamsters, and Guinea Pigs

These nocturnal rodents are a little kid's favorite. They're small, cute, and pretty active, and they enjoy burrowing, which makes them fun to watch. Take note that a hamster plus a wheel equals an all-night running party. If you bring home a boy and a girl hamster, be ready for a million babies, as hamsters multiply as fast as "Gremlins." That, or they will sometimes fight to the death and kill each other, which can make for an interesting scene with your screaming toddler. Make sure to keep the hamster cage in a place where you will most likely find an unsightly crime scene first, before your toddler does.

You might find guinea pigs adorable, unless you've had one squeak all night in your bedroom. I'm not exaggerating when I say they squeak *all night,* and they're quite loud. They're also not particularly friendly (think bunny rabbit), and they have pretty big teeth (again, think bunny rabbit). However, many kids in 4-H adore them and enjoy taking care of them until the time of their local fair.

Bunny Rabbits

While rabbits are adorable creatures, they're not commonly great house pets. An important factor is that rabbits are nervous and typically don't enjoy being held. They will shake with fright, kick, bite, and struggle to be released. This fragile animal is also quick and can be hard to catch. It's amazing how good they are at hiding. Think again if you are looking for a pet your child can cuddle with.

Rats

The best-kept secret is that rats make wonderful pets for children. They're easily tamed and become attached to their owner, taking on their owner's temperament at times. They're pretty low maintenance but like to exercise and play. Some owners swear their rat comes when called by name. Rats are intelligent, as well, with males being notably lazier than the females. With a life span of 2 to 3 years, the commitment is pretty short-lived for these nocturnal love bugs. Who knew?!?!

Reptiles

Reptiles are for the more mature pet owner. They're relatively easy to care for, if you can stomach feeding them live crickets (who will chirp loudly until eaten) and/or mice (who will squeak loudly until eaten). They usually require a sun lamp to keep them warm, regardless of the temperature in your home, so if you're light sensitive, these may not be good pets for you.

While geckoes and some breeds of lizards are relatively harmless, I can't think of anything more frightening than finding a snake slithering up into my baby's crib. Know your state's safety guidelines for owning reptiles and take extra precautionary measures. Or, play it extra safe and wait till your child is in high school before starting your cobra farm.

Turtles, both water and land varieties, are interesting pets, but again, they require a lot of care. Water turtles are susceptible to disease, so make sure your child washes his hands directly after handling the turtle. Also, water turtles scratch on the glass walls of their aquariums while swimming, which can be annoying to sensitive ears. Desert tortoises hibernate from November to around March, making them a perfect half-a-year pet. (The best part—you don't have to worry about securing a pet sitter during your winter holiday!). Turtles are also yummy snacks for crows and other flying predators, however, so be wary if they're kept outside during the summer months. Most reptiles will not hold your child's attention for very long, as they're not the most exciting creatures for a toddler to watch.

Outdoor Animals

If you are fortunate enough to have outdoor animals and livestock, such as cows, sheep, pigs, horses, chickens, and turkeys, just take note of your child's allergies and whether he has an aversion to an animal's dander or poop. Chickens and turkeys are messy birds, so clean their coops often, and make sure you wash your baby's hands if he's helped you gather eggs. If you take the proper precautionary actions to ensure that your animals and children are safe, you will most likely avoid any sensory issues with your kids living in a farm environment. Now, if you can only get that rooster to crow later in the morning!

Stay-at-Home Mom (or Dad!)

"Try to be quiet and still in those moments that tend to over-whelm and cause confusion. I have found throughout my journey (as a mom and occupational therapist) that it is when the gap between our inner knowing and outer actions becomes too wide that we must return to the basics—a soft chair, a cold glass of water, and the wisdom in our hearts."

—DR ANGELA N. HISSONG, OTR/L, CAPS

Being a stay-at-home mom is wonderful, but it is also a considerable amount of work. Taking care of a newborn is exhausting and can completely deplete a person, especially if you don't have any help. It is easy to lose your identity as you're catering to a baby's every need, and moms with difficult or challenging babies can be beyond exhaustion. If you're starting to think that 30 days without food and water on CBS's "Survivor" looks like a cakewalk for pansies, than you most likely need some much-deserved rest and relaxation. But how could you possibly leave your angel for one second? You can, and you will, eventually.

Spouse/Partner Takes a Turn

I, for one, am extremely auditory sensitive. If my husband is watching loud TV and my son is playing a noisy game on the computer, I have to go outside for some peace. It's too much, and I can't think. So I'm often on walk-the-dog duty, which includes picking up poop. At least I'm outside, and it's quiet. I can think about nothing but the trees and look in other peoples' houses and wonder how they live. It is oddly soothing to see families making diner and watching TV throughout the neighborhood. Are there any duties you can do outside the home? Do you take your clothes to a Laundromat? Even that can be a getaway while your spouse is on baby duty. Want to take the lawn mower for a spin? Why don't you put yourself on yard duty on Saturday morning, while your spouse makes breakfast with your baby? Why don't you take the car in for an oil change and explore the surrounding area on foot, while you're waiting. Again, be creative. Try something new, or do something that you wouldn't usually do. It doesn't have to be a cooking class to be an outing.

MOM TIP: Another thing I have found that works wonders is to have an activity planned or a special movie in the DVD player for when your significant other gets home from work. It can be less daunting for your husband if there is already something in motion when he walks in and gets to be the "King of Finger Painting" or, upon his entrance, a much-anticipated children's movie is in the DVD player and he only has to push "play." Look, there is specially made popcorn for him, too! You can slip out the door for a mani-pedi and be back before the end credits roll.

Parents, In-Laws, and Family Members

If your family lives nearby, ask if there's a time they could get some "alone" time with your baby or children. Grandparents love to spoil the children, and they enjoy getting to be with them without you around. Take advantage of these glorious, free babysitters if they're available to you. They will be glad you did.

For those of you with in-laws who live five states away, get on the phone and beg for a visit. If they're able to schedule trips out to see you, ask them to come as often as they can and talk to them about having quality alone time with the children. Most of them will take you up on this offer, as having this special time with their grandchildren is priceless.

Are there any other family members nearby? An aunt? A cousin? Someone you trust and who could perhaps use some babysitting practice to prepare for having her own children? Family isn't just for Thanksgiving dinners! Even if you have to drive a town or two over to get your baby to her house, you can find a local theater or explore the main street while she watches your baby for a few hours. As a loving aunt myself, I enjoy offering up a Friday evening or Saturday afternoon to help out. I always enjoy being with my nephew, and I know it's nice for his parents to get out and have some "alone time." My significant other and I have even gone over for "baby duty" while his mommy and daddy painted their hallway! We didn't want little baby handprints on the freshly painted walls.

Friends and Other Mothers (or Fathers!)

If you have any friends with children, whether they're the same age as your baby or not, you can start a babysitting-bartering plan with them. You can take their children on Monday, and they can take your children on Wednesday. Moms are fantastic babysitters, and they are usually understanding if your plans change at the last minute, due to a baby coming down with a virus during the night.

Don't have any friends with kids? What about that lady you liked that was in your mommy yoga group? Or, you can join some mommy groups online and get to know a few of the mothers. This isn't something you need to jump into. Take your time, and really get to know some of the other mothers. Do they have the same parenting mindset as you? Are their children clean and groomed? Or, are they at least attended to? (Some children are extremely messy, and no mom can keep them clean for 5 minutes.) How does this mom speak to her children? Is she respectful and courteous, but firm? Does she set boundaries? Do your homework when looking for a mom or two that you want to start a baby-watching co-op with. This may be a relationship that extends into the future of your children. You will be sitting in the high-school bleachers, watching your little boys dominate the field together. Yes, your baby is going to grow up eventually.

How Often?

Start with once a week and ease into one or two planned activities out of the home by yourself, once you've gotten used to short breaks.

What to Do? Who Am I Again?

- Take a bath. Get some glorious-smelling bath salts or essential oils to sprinkle in. If you can still hear your baby crying while you're in the bath, this does not count as a relaxing 15 minutes to yourself.

- Take a yoga class.

- Take a walk.

- Get a facial or give yourself one in your bedroom with the door closed while your partner watches the children.

- Get a mani-pedi or give yourself one.

- Read a book—and not one for your child. Read one just for you! A trashy romance novel or an engaging biography can provide a welcome escape and give your senses a reprieve.

- Make a lunch date with an old friend.

- Reconnect with high-school friends on Facebook. Warning: Ex-boyfriends will surface and try to rekindle an old flame. Many a marriage and relationship have been ruined by this newfound social networking device—so be wary. There may be a reason it didn't work out all those years ago. We recommend looking at your old friends' baby photos, instead!

- Start a blog. If you have an interest or passion for gardening, sewing, or a topic others might want to connect about, share your information and your perspective. You might find a connection or a voice inside you, yearning to get out.

Mommy Goes to Work
(Pumping, Guilt, and Alone Time)

"Multitasking is out. Multisensory is in!"

—Jackie Linder Olson

Let's face it—while life can be wonderful, it can also be stressful. We all have endless tasks to accomplish and most likely get more done in a day than people used to get done in a week. Why? Because we are expected to, and because we can! Remember when it used to be that the father went to work, while the mother stayed home, cleaning house and making pies? Well, more mothers are in the work force now than ever before. Either they have a passion for their career, or they need to help the family financially and they're working hard. While we can't all be "every woman," like the Whitney Houston song says, we can find a healthy balance between work and home life. We find this combination is easier on a parent (dads too!) if you take your own sensory needs into consideration.

Daily Sensory Overload

Does your typical day involve rising before the sun to ensure the kids' lunches are packed and to finish that last-minute presentation your boss requested, before rushing the baby to the sitter's house and stopping to pick up your dry cleaning on the way into work? While you sit in traffic, with road rage brewing in the cars around you, do you think to yourself that your day is just getting started, and you have 9 hours of grueling duties ahead of you before you can pick up your baby and attempt to make it to your son's soccer practice? You're not alone. Even those of you who love your jobs find it tough to get it all done in a typical day. It may sound simple, but we'd like to remind you to breathe. In. Out. Take a moment during your drive to breathe. Slow down your internal systems and focus.

Some things to consider that might be adding to your stress and discomfort may be that your senses need to be taken care of. For example, are the air-conditioning ducts at work blowing rancid air into your office? This can be extremely difficult on your respiratory system and cause eye and olfactory irritation. If you spend your days in a cubicle, are you constantly bombarded with the noise of other people on the phone, the fax machine, the copy machine, printers running, and an overall hubbub of organized chaos? Your sensory system never gets a break in that environment, and it would benefit you to take a brisk stroll outside during your lunch break, even if you can only spare 15 minutes. Do you stare at a computer all day? Are the fluorescent lights at work giving you headaches? Is there a loudspeaker echoing throughout your workplace all day long? These things can wear you down, and you may need a sensory pick-me-up.

If your place of work doesn't already have an employee lounge, you should check your local labor laws to find out if one is required. While this room doesn't have to have Pottery Barn furnishings, it should be a peaceful place where you can unwind. Some guys might find it relaxing to catch 15 minutes of a hockey game on their break, which is fine, if that works for you. Others might need 15 minutes to read a book or enjoy some soft music. If you find that you're bombarded by other employees during this break, you should talk to a manager about making the break room a quiet space. Think spa environment. Everyone is there to have a time-out. Dish about the hot guy in accounting and what happened last night on "Desperate Housewives" another time.

Your desk, or your office, is most likely someplace that you spend a good amount of your time. Decorate it accordingly. While it's common for mothers to want to use every inch of their workspace as a shrine to their baby and/or family, limit this space to a few favorite pictures. When you use the "less is more" philosophy, you can get more accomplished during the day and keep your senses in check if you keep the clutter to a minimum. Not that baby photos are clutter, but when you add in paperwork, phone, computer, pens, safety clips, and so on, it all starts to add up and take up space not only on your desk but in your visual space.

Some offices allow candles. If a candle helps calm you, and you don't set your office on fire, fabulous. Hang paintings or posters of inspirational quotes or a tranquil ocean picture in your line of sight to remind you to slow down and breathe.

Take into consideration if your boss's expectations of you are too high. Do you have so many tasks on your to-do list that it's impossible to ever complete them? Or, are you too hard on yourself and expecting too much out of yourself in an average day?

Pumping at Work

Have you decided to breastfeed when you go back to work? Good for you! Pumping sure makes it a heck of a lot easier than it used to be. If you have your own office, great! Lock the door and pump away. Pick a time when you can ignore the phones and take a few minutes to yourself, and be careful that you're not flashing the offices across the street from you. Some moms look at a photo of their baby while pumping and swear it helps the milk pump easier.

If you don't have an office to pump in, fret not. Bathrooms are a fine place to pump, and many mothers find being by a sink convenient. I know women who have pumped in all sorts of places, from their cars to a supply closet. When there's a pump, there's a way! Try to keep a healthy mindset, stay focused, and know that you're doing the best you can do for your baby.

"You" Time

Just because you are working does not mean you have to forego your right to have some alone time. In fact, you might need it even more, since you don't give your sensory systems as many breaks throughout the day. If you are a gym rat, go ahead and schedule that spin class after work before heading home. Your body and mind will be healthier, and you'll be able to tend to your baby with a clearer perspective.

Maybe you need an extra hour each morning to meditate or a few hours on the weekend for a pottery class. It's amazing how much more you can give when you're fulfilled. As a martyr myself, I will run myself ragged trying to take care of everyone else. When I'm finally forced to have a facial by a well-meaning friend, I feel so rejuvenated that I'm a better and more attentive mother. We have to remember to take care of ourselves too and not feel guilty if we're gone a large percentage of the day. The important thing is that your child is taken care of and loved and that the time you do spend together is quality time.

Be *Home* at Home!

A few things I've found to make my time at home quality time with my child is to get as much done as I can before I get home. There is nothing worse for your little one than to finally have you home, and you have other things to tend to besides him.

Turn off your cell phone, stop checking emails, and do not log onto Facebook until your child is asleep (not just in bed, but asleep!). Everything else can wait during those few precious hours with your family, no matter how important you think you are.

Once a week, pay your bills at lunchtime instead of going out. With online bill pay, there is no reason to be writing checks when you get home from work and your child is waiting for your undivided attention.

Leave your work at work, or in your car, until your child is asleep. Work has had your attention all day, and your child needs you when you're at home. Also, you do not want to wake up down the road and wonder why you missed his childhood—you will not get a second chance!

Reconnecting

After a long day at work and daycare, you and your baby will need to reconnect. If you pick your child up from daycare, spend a moment chatting with the providers about your child's day. Take a look at the artwork your toddler made and maybe examine a new toy your child is excited about. Once you and your child are in the car, maybe sing a silly song, or sing in an opera voice really badly and ask if your child thinks you're a good singer. Make the car ride home enjoyable for both of you and use the time to reconnect.

At times, your child may be emotional and have some difficulty reconnecting after a long or stressful day. He may be angry with you and show you by hitting you or pushing you away. Or maybe he's sad and he'll cry, turning his back on you and clinging to the nanny or day-care provider. While this may be hurtful to you, or frustrating, or annoying, take a step back and remember that as the adult and parent, it is your responsibility to work on reconnecting. Let your child know that you understand he's frustrated or angry and that you wish you could spend every waking second with him, but that is just not possible. Let your child pout in the car for a bit if he needs to, and then maybe pretend to see a wild purple elephant in the road. Ask if your child sees the wild purple elephant too and ask if you should call a zookeeper? Eventually, your child will most likely crack a smile and start to warm up to you again. It can be a lot of work to be creative and pull your child back into your world, but it will be worth it for you to be able to enjoy each other's company for the few hours before bedtime.

You may have to go through the process again once Daddy (or your partner) gets home, but the bonds between child and parent need constant nurturing. It will be good for all parties involved.

CHAPTER SIX

Growing Up
(2 to 3 Years)

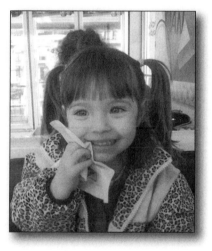

First trip to Disneyland for this little princess!
HARMONY, 2 YEARS OLD

Your Not-So-Terrible 2-Year-Old

BY THIS TIME, YOU KNOW IF YOUR CHILD IS A RUNNER OR A CLINGER. YOU'VE either been dashing around after your quick little guy, or you carry him on your hip constantly, like a mother monkey. While both toddler types have their pros and cons, it is safe to say that most toddlers like to assert their authority. This is a natural phase in your child's life, where he will try and control his environment. Here are some tips that could help.

Sense of Humor

While not necessarily a sense, this life-saving defense mechanism will often get you through the day with your child. Parenting is funny. By now you're used to changing poopy diapers and cleaning up mucus, vomit, and every other bodily fluid. Before embarking on the years of toddlerhood, give your funny bone a tune-up, because potty training and a mountain of fresh challenges are around the corner.

People such as Ray Romano and Bill Cosby have made multimillion-dollar careers out of the things their kids say. I keep a list of some of the particularly humorous lines my son has said to put in his scrap-book. You will forget these gems in a few years, so it's nice to have them in a safe place to look back on and get more laughs out of them.

Being silly at times will help you through your toddler's outbursts and will help you keep your sanity.

Thick Skin

As a parent, you will need to have a moderately thick skin, otherwise known as not getting offended easily. Your little baby will grow into a child, who, at some point, will tell you she hates you, you're ruining her life, and that you're by far the worst parent in the world. I knew this would happen, but I was shocked it happened so early. Being that it was entirely out of context and I'm pretty sure he had no idea what it meant, I was able to shake it off easily. As my son grows, however, and I know he's saying things like that to hurt me, it's a bit harder to swallow. I do, however, recommend that you take it for what it is—your child expressing his anger—and know that it will pass. If you draw too much attention to it, he will know it's a soft spot with you and will take advantage at the next available occasion. What I do is say, "I hear that you are angry, but it's not okay to say that to Mommy," and I'll either give him a few minutes to calm down or I'll put him in a time-out (or a "time-in," as they're now called).

Remember that the toddler years prep you for when they are teenagers.

Which Sense?

There is no way to decipher which sense is the most important overall, but there will be senses that your toddler relies on more than others. Some children are very visual, some gravitate toward sounds, some seek touch, and, on the alternate end of the spectrum, others avoid certain sounds and smells. How do you sift through what is important and what is an underlying behavior or condition that your child may be secretly suffering from? Kids are amazing adapters. Our little magicians can hide a sensory problem, such as an aversion to sound; however, it could resurface later in life as a serious condition. If an auditory issue is not addressed, your child could have problems later, with speech pronunciation, hearing in the classroom, or blocking out noises like a clock ticking in class or understanding safety rules. Here you'll find some tips and guides to help decipher if your toddler is having a sensory-processing issue or if it is something else entirely. As a parent or caregiver, it is your responsibility to be a sensory detective and examine the clues that you will find by means of observation.

Sensory Issue or Allergies (or Intolerance)

If your child is cranky and aggravated every time she's at a certain park or she cries when she's around your neighbor's dog, see what other signs she's showing during these difficult times. Is her nose running? Does she have itchy eyes? Is she always a bit more difficult and bossy when she's in the laundry room downstairs? Is there mold that she could be allergic to? Nowadays, a lot of people have allergies. If your toddler has itchy eyes or dark circles under her eyes, acts as if she has a cold, has a skin rash, or has developed a chronic cough from postnasal drip, please have your child tested for allergies.

Also, something parents are becoming more aware of is if their child has food intolerance to items such as gluten, dairy products, or soy. Some children can't digest these items, and it shows itself as erratic behavior after eating one of these items. Other children might be slug-

133

gish after eating an item they have intolerance to, and still others may have increased anxiety and are unable to focus. For example, my son has intolerance to gluten, and once we eliminated gluten from his diet, his anxiety decreased considerably. We eliminated milk, and his teacher has said that he is more alert and can focus better. Food intolerances can go unnoticed and undiagnosed for several years but are garnering more and more attention as more is learned about these mysterious intolerances. If you suspect that your child may have a food intolerance, you should speak with her pediatrician and get a recommendation to work with a nutritionist who specializes in such matters.

Sensory or Behavioral Issue?

In their toddler years, most children are going to exhibit some behaviors that you as a parent may not like. Some of this will stem from typical development, some of it may be due to an underlying sensory issue, and some may truly be a behavioral issue. How to tell all of these apart sometimes takes a professional eye to determine, but you can start by asking yourself a few questions.

When your child is happy, has slept well, is well fed, and seems to be having a good day, does she transition from one activity to the next without a major meltdown? If her sandwich is not cut in half the way she usually likes, does she roll with it? If you are driving along and realize you forgot her favorite toy for the car, does she play with something different, or can she be distracted by singing songs?

If your child suddenly begins to throw a tantrum and you cannot figure out why, then it could be caused by a sensory issue. Sensory needs are hard to see all of the time, and you have to take into consideration the environment, how much sleep your child has had, how loud is the ambient environment, has her routine been changed, and have you been trying something new with her. Every child will be slightly hesitant sometimes when trying something new, but if she always refuses to touch anything that is sticky, gooey, or mushy, she might have some tactile defensiveness going on.

If you are in the grocery store and your child is fussy and you cannot calm her down, she could be bothered by the fluorescent lighting or the volume of the music in the store. If your child suddenly throws herself on the floor because you told her she could not have a candy bar, then this may strictly be a behavioral issue. When a child throws tantrums when you tell her "no" and when you tell her she cannot play with her little sister because she is being too rough, or when she gets upset and screams and cries when you turn off her favorite TV show, these scenarios typically turn out to be behavioral in nature. Again, if you are having difficulty managing your child and you think it could have something to do with her sensory systems not processing information correctly and/or efficiently, contact your pediatrician and get a referral to see an occupational therapist in your area.

Sensory Issue or Hunger?

Is your child out of energy? Is he cranky because he's hungry? Is your child's blood sugar low? I have always had to eat snacks throughout the day to avoid fainting. I was borderline hypoglycemic as a child and had gestational diabetes while I was pregnant. It wasn't until my mid-30s when I learned more about proper nutrition and gave up gluten, dairy, and soy that I was actually able to regulate my blood sugar. A natural blood-sugar regulator is cinnamon, but don't make yourself some cinnamon toast with processed sugar and expect it to work. Sugar, fructose, corn syrup, and all chemical and synthetic forms of sugar are known to produce insulin, which deregulates your blood-sugar levels.

If your baby or child is hungry, it may cause other sensory systems to not function properly, and your child might throw tantrums for the most asinine reasons. Make sure you have (watered down) 100% real fruit juices available and some snacks like nuts, bananas and apples, and Cheerios—anything your child is able to eat to keep her blood-sugar levels higher than the danger zone.

Sensory Issue or Separation Anxiety?

Some children may have a tantrum or throw themselves down on the floor and scream bloody murder if their parent leaves, or, better yet, attempts to leave. If your child holds onto you like a cat above water as you head for the door, then he could be demonstrating separation anxiety. Some children who know that their parent is getting ready to leave will suddenly come down with a stomachache or some other ailment to try to keep the parent from leaving. If your child sheds big tears and makes a dramatic scene, make sure that you're kind but firm and that you give him reassurance that you will return soon. Never sneak out and leave your child to avoid a tantrum. That will only make your departure worse in the future, and you will ruin your trusting relationship with your child. Instead, have a fun activity planned for your babysitter or caregiver to do with your toddler after you leave. Most often, your child will calm down and enjoy himself while you are gone. This is good practice for your toddler to learn to regulate his internal systems.

If your child is experiencing separation anxiety while he's at the park, being dropped off at daycare, or at a dance class, perhaps your child needs a few proprioceptive squeezes from you and some positive encouragement. A few shoulder squeezes or a deep-pressure hug will help your child regulate his proprioceptive system and may allow him to separate more easily. If he seeks that pressure, perhaps a sensational T-shirt from Fun and Function would be helpful, or a weighted vest to help calm your child down during transitions.

We recommend working with your pediatrician, psychologist, or occupational therapist if you feel that the separation anxiety is atypical and is not something your child is growing out of.

Sensory Issue or Stubbornness

Let's face it—like adults, some toddlers are more stubborn than others. "Set in their ways" is a term that is usually reserved for the elderly, but we've found that there are toddlers who are set in their ways, too. Does your child only like you to play a game one way? Does your child only want food prepared one way? Once your child learns a new skill, is there only ONE right way to do it? If this is just stubbornness and not obsession, then your child may either grow out of his ways once he releases some of his control over his environment, or he may just be one of those people who are not flexible.

A way to tell if your child is having a sensory-processing issue and is not just being stubborn is if you are not able to coax your child with your usual bag of tricks to even try something new. If you prepare a peanut butter and jelly sandwich for your child on a new type of bread and she goes ballistic, this is probably just stubbornness, and she will eventually give in and eat the new bread. A child with SPD will not give in and won't be able to tolerate either the smell or the texture of the new bread. Another example of a sensory issue could be if your child always complains that things are too tight, too cold, too sticky, etcetera. "Too" something is a small indicator that maybe there are some underlying sensory difficulties, and contacting an occupational therapist in your area can help you determine if your child truly does have sensory issues.

Sensory Issue or Exhaustion?

A toddler's schedule can be as cram-packed as that of a busy CEO. Counting bugs, having a playdate, and joining Mommy on errands can wipe a kid out. Make sure that if your child is fussy and irritable, you consider how much sleep she got last night, if she had a good nap, or if it is getting close to bedtime.

One of my friends thought her daughter was having sensory problems, but it turned out she just needed more sleep. After adjusting her bedtime to be one hour earlier in the evening, her daughter's sensory issues disappeared. As we've mentioned before, a proper amount of good sleep is crucial to your toddler's well-being.

Communicating with Your Child

Britt and I are both talkers, and our significant others are able to completely tune us out. Your toddler has most likely developed that same talent, especially if you're a constant talker. Eventually, your words all run together, and she's able to go about her business of gluing sticks, chasing bugs, and exploring the world while you shout orders, beg her to mind, and threaten to throw all her toys into the wastebasket. If you find your voice falling on deaf ears, there are a few things you can do to turn the situation around. Remember, you're in this for the long haul and will need to invest some time into retraining your toddler to hear you.

First of all, does your child have an auditory sensitivity issue? Does she turn and look at you when you call her name? Does your toddler startle with loud noises, or is she oblivious to sounds such as the doorbell? Does your child get upset when you vacuum or use the blender? Does your child cringe when your older children play their video games too loud? You may need to check with your pediatrician and possibly a specialist to make sure your child's ears are in tip-top shape. While my pediatrician told me my son's ears were "fine," a specialist later told me his ear canals were clogged, and we had to use steroids for 3 days to help clean them out. He explained that my son could hear the equivalent of Charlie Brown's teacher, "Wah, wah, wah, wah, wah, wah." So, if in doubt, ask your pediatrician to recommend an ear specialist to be sure that your toddler can actually hear you.

Less Is More

After ruling out a medical condition, listen to yourself talk. Do you go on and on and on and on and on about the same thing? Do you repeat yourself one hundred times that the clothes need to be taken out the dryer, or that you're the only one who does the laundry? Some people don't talk much at all, and some talk way more than they need to. Your child doesn't know and is learning about what words to pick out of everything you say that might be important to and/or directed at her. Choose your words wisely.

There are different ways to speak to your toddler, and you may as well start the two-way street of communication now. This will be a valuable investment that will pay off later on.

When you ask your toddler to perform a task, get down to his level and look him in the eyes. Keep your directions on par with his age and skill level. For example, get down on your knees and tell Johnny, "It's clean-up time. Start by putting your trains into their box." Don't talk about how he has to learn to clean up his toys or about how you're not his maid or how, after cleaning up toys, you're going to the grocery store and then to pick up the dry cleaning. Focus. Be clear, polite, and respectful, and then get out of there. If Johnny is too busy playing with his trains and ignores you, tap him lightly on the shoulder. When he looks at you, repeat yourself. Johnny may not like hearing that it is time to put the toys away, so maybe you can say, "Johnny, you may play with the trains for two more minutes and then we're going to clean up." Give Johnny 2 minutes to finish his thought process and transition to putting the trains away. You may then need to physically help Johnny put the trains away. Make it a game if possible. "Johnny, can you put away all the blue trains, and I'll put away the red ones!"

TIME. Who has all this extra time to coax your toddler into cleaning up her toys? We suggest that you make the time. Maybe you don't get everything done in one day that you would like, but investing time in positive communication with your child will make a huge difference in the quality of your days to come. When you put in the time with your toddler, you're showing her respect, building trust, and creating solid communication.

Stop!

Toddlers are not able to think and then move their bodies as quickly as adults. If you say to Sally, "Stop that this instant," it make take a few moments for Sally to process what you want her to stop doing and then to get her body to stop. If you want to see how quickly your child can react to the verbal request to stop, play the music-freeze game. Explain to your toddler that you're going to play a dance game and you're going to freeze like statues when the music stops. You may have to show her what you mean and then play the game together. Dance, dance, then shut off the music and say, "Freeze." You may find that your toddler takes a few moments to think, then stop, and then freeze into a pose. It is not an instant process. Your little one's hearing reflexes will get stronger and her gross-motor reflexes will get faster as she grows up. For the time being, when you have a request, give your toddler time to process it before repeating yourself again and again. Every time you vocalize another request, she has to start processing all over again.

Screaming, Shouting, and Yelling

When you scream at your toddler, neither you nor your toddler wins. You both end up upset, and you've done nothing more than waste your time on an ineffectual form of communication. Screaming and getting irrational only creates a negative situation, and it will take more time to do whatever you're trying to accomplish. Do you want your child to hurry up? Well, if you have all of her items ready to go and she's not able to move as quickly as you'd like, then you're better off helping your child and saving a lesson on rushing for when you're not in such a rush. If your child is a dilly dallier, then no amount of screaming is going to encourage her to move at a quicker pace. You will have to move your toddler along by helping with her shoes or gathering up her books and carrying her out the door. If she's disagreeable to this, then give her the option to move at a faster pace on her own. Perhaps suggest a "race" to get out the door. Who can be ready to go first and be waiting by the door? Whoever gets his shoes on the fastest gets to pick the music in the car! For your sanity, be creative and think of ways to make listening to you fun. If your toddler thinks that Mommy or Daddy will be saying something interesting and I might miss out if I'm not listening, then your words will become far more valuable.

It's a Jungle in Here

Can your child hear you and literally be able to process what you've said? If you're in a noisy area, such as a shopping center or a baseball game where there is a loudspeaker blaring, your child is not going to be able to process you telling her to wipe her nose. At times when your toddler is already processing large amounts of information, such as noises, activity (such as baseball players running), and a soft rain falling, while simultaneously having to navigate up into the bleachers as she holds a bag of peanuts, she's literally not going to be able to turn everything off and focus on what you are saying. Help your child to do what you would like her to do, and get her attention when she's seated and able to focus on your words.

The Silent Treatment

I've seen some parents ignore their child's tantrum or turn away from their child when they ask for something over and over again. I'm not sure if the theory is that if you ignore it, it will go away, or if you ignore it, you're not giving it any attention, but from what we've seen, this method can be pretty ineffective. Your child may throw a tantrum because of a need, and they're asking you questions because they need repetition, attention, and feedback to be able to learn and grow. I know it can be tiresome and often a pain, but repeating an answer to your toddler rather than ignoring her is teaching her that you care about her and her needs. We're not saying you have to cater to your toddler's every whim, but even saying, "Mommy needs some quiet time right now" acknowledges your child, and, hopefully, she will stop pushing your buttons while you recollect yourself.

"Zen thoughts" and the silent treatment are not the same. When my toddler was driving me up the wall and making me really bonkers, I started saying, "You need to practice being quiet right now." For example, it started in the car on the freeway. I would say, "Okay, quiet time for five miles. You need to be silent for Mommy while I drive." This was an extremely challenging task for my child, and he was often unsuccessful, but I'm glad we kept working on it because now, when I get on the freeway, he starts reading a book or playing his DS and it is quiet. I cherish those moments as much as the big smiles and kisses I get from him.

You can also help your child quiet himself, a valuable skill with life-long benefits. If both you and your toddler have had a busy morning and you're both at your wits' end, have a snack and hydrate, and then have "Zen time." Snuggle up on the couch and read books (or look at pictures). Practice breathing deeply and stretching together. Get out your gardening gear and turn over some dirt (to get ready for that garden you may or may not get around to planting). Pick a name for this type of time together. Quiet time. Zen time. Peaceful-thoughts time. Pink-bunny time. Whatever works for you and your toddler. Again, make time for this type of relaxation. In our hectic world, if your child doesn't learn to relax and enjoy being a toddler, it is going to be harder for him to calm his body and regulate himself for years to come.

Choices: My Way or My Way

We know you've been told this a million times before, and we're going to say it, as well: "When you say 'no' to your child, you have to mean it." 'No' does not mean 'maybe.' 'No' does not mean that when you cry and scream for 45 minutes, I will give in and give it to you. 'No' has got to be the final word. If you have to cave in, make sure you add a condition, such as, "I will reconsider after you have cleaned your room," or "I will talk to Daddy about it, and we will decide together if you brush your teeth for two minutes without whining." This is imperative in raising your child and in curbing countless arguments.

Now, here is a wonderful way to get your child to do what you want and to have him be happy about it. I call it the "My Way or My Way Choice." Once you have firmly established that 'no' means 'no,' you may start the My Way or My Way Choice method.

Give your child two choices, making your preference the most desirable choice A, but make sure you're also comfortable with option B. For example, if you lay out two school outfits for your child to choose from, make sure you're happy with either outfit. Here are some situational choice examples:

- *You're at a toy store, and you need to get a birthday present for your niece. This can be hard on your child or children for obvious reasons.*

    Scenario A. Select two items for your child to choose from, such as two stuffed animals or two puzzles. You can pick out two items under 10 dollars, and let your child make the choice of which one to buy. This way she's part of the process!

    Scenario B. You can let the reward for helping out be the choice your child makes. For instance, you could let her select either a Barbie doll or an Easy-Bake Oven for her cousin. Then say, "Wow, you were so helpful! Would you like to choose your reward? You could have some extra TV time or some extra time on the computer when we get home—you pick."

What's the Point Again?

What you're establishing with your child is that *(a)* 'No' means 'no.' *(b)* He has control over making choices. *(c)* If he makes the right choice, he will be rewarded. And by having two choices for your child that you can live with and he will be happy with, as well, you're building the foundation for a peaceful and successful relationship. Spinach or broccoli is not a choice your toddler will always be happy with, but, again, a choice gives him some control over eating his vegetables. Maybe the choice is in the reward he gets for eating his vegetables—he can pick a dessert or a game for the family to play together after he eats them.

If you're constantly telling your child exactly what to do, you're going to create resentment with your little one and create more battles over control. Your toddler is going to want to assert his independence, and not giving him choices will only infuriate his natural tendencies. Also, you want your child to start understanding choices because all of life is choices. At some point, your child is going to go off into the world and have to think for himself. What greater gift than sending him out of the nest equipped with solid decision-making skills?

Inspiring your toddler to think for herself, make good choices, and get things done is the name of the game. We're not asking you to debate what to have for dinner every night with your toddler. Again, you narrow it down to two choices that she gets to pick. If she does not make a choice, or if she has a fit, then you take the choices away. "Okay, now it's Mommy's choice. We're having chicken nuggets and corn." As with saying no, you have to stick with your choice.

I Changed My Mind!

Everyone is going to change her mind at times. What if you tell Melissa she can't have a half-hour of computer time, and then you want to talk to your best friend on the phone about her recent engagement, and then you actually *want* Melissa occupied on the computer. It's all right to tell Melissa that you have thought about it and that if she puts away her dolls nicely on her bed, then she may use the computer for half an hour. Your child will be thrilled with the compromise, but make sure you don't make this a habit too often or your word will lose its value. Again, the point is to curb whining, tantrums, and negative behaviors, so if you're wishy-washy with the rules, you're leaving yourself open for issues to develop. If your toddler believes that she can whine, scream, kick, or use a negative behavior to get you to cave in, you're toast. So change your mind from time to time, but still make it about doing something good and getting rewarded for positive behavior.

Potty Training

There is a certain scare factor in transitioning a child from diapers to pull-ups to big-kid pants. I have encountered many situations where I have helped families look at potty training from a sensory point of view. You have to look at the situation from the perspective of a child, as you know your child's needs, likes, and dislikes. You can take a step back and look at the sensory factors going into the act of potty training to find the underlying reason why your child may be having a difficult time with this task. Most importantly, relax.

Is Your Child Ready?

A big mistake parents make is trying to force a child to potty train before he's ready. Are you about to go on a trip with your sister and her kids for a week at Disneyland? Your child is going to be far more interested in playing with his cousins and seeing Mickey Mouse than potty training. Wait until after your trip to start.

I tell the parents that I work with to try and look for cues that your child has to go to the bathroom, even if he is not able to verbally communicate this to you. Watch his body language, practice sitting on the toilet when you think it is close to time for him to urinate or have a bowel movement, and consider using a picture schedule with your child. Monitor times of the day when your child usually has a bowel movement, and take note of how often he needs to use the restroom after he eats and drinks. Most clues are subtle, but if your child is taking off his dirty diaper and handing it to you, he's more than ready.

Another thing to note is that it is usually easier for children to learn how to urinate in the toilet first and then worry about working on having a bowel movement. Once you can get the child on a routine of using the potty, he becomes much more willing to have a bowel movement on the potty, as well.

Are You Ready?

One of the biggest elements in potty training is you. You have to be consistent in bringing your child into the restroom periodically. You are going to have to clean up any accidents on the living-room rug and around the toilet seat. You are going to have to remind your child to go potty before you leave to run your errands. You are going to have to find a bathroom while you are in the grocery store with your toddler. You are going to have to prevent his little hands from going into the tampon disposal bin in the public restroom (it happened to me once, and I'll never be the same!).

Are you nervous about this natural developmental milestone? If so, maybe you need to relax a little bit and understand that this, like any other milestone, is going to happen. Your child is going to become potty trained, and it can be either a pleasant experience or a struggle. The choice is almost completely up to you, and the rest is up to your toddler.

Where to Start?

Have you been talking about potty training with your little one? There are many books for kids on potty training that are fun and informative. Surely this will start a dialog between the two of you. There are potty-training DVDs such as, "Bear in the Big Blue House—Potty Time with Bear" by Disney. This was a big hit with my son, who is a visual learner. There are potty-training kits on teaching your child to potty train in one day. While these might be helpful, do not put pressure on yourself or your child to make this transition in such a short time frame.

You will need a potty to start—either a portable one for toddlers or the kind you can place onto the adult potty. Your child may need a stool if you are using the bigger potty, as he will want to place his feet on the stool to help with balance and for pushing on when having a bowel movement. You'll need an extra potty in the car. I didn't take anyone's advice on this, which I quickly regretted. My son was terrified of public restrooms at first and wanted "his" potty while we were out and about. Upon getting a second potty at the dollar store for the back of my minivan, mobile potty training became a cinch.

Some kids are motivated and enjoy being a part of picking out a cushy cartoon-character toilet seat. Other children enjoy looking at a special book or playing a game while they sit on the potty.

Reward System

A reward system will help inspire your child and help you keep track of when your child is successful at using the potty or keeping her pull-up dry. It can be a great resource to use a sticker chart or a reward system to help your child understand that if she is successful in the task, she is rewarded with something she enjoys, such as stickers, a trip to the park, a game, or the like.

Some parents are using the "potty party" method (where you reward the child with a "party" every time she uses a "big-girl potty"), but we have gotten mixed reviews from parents. Toddlers who enjoy big parties and a lot of attention might be delighted with a potty party, while a more sensitive and introverted child might find a potty party embarrassing and overwhelming. Cater potty training to your child, just as you would any other task.

Sensory Potty Training

Many times, it takes an occupational therapist's skilled eye to see what your child's specific sensory needs are, which can in turn help you muscle through this difficult time. Here are a few things to consider when tackling the task of potty training:

- Is your child sensitive to the cold toilet seat?
- Is your child uncomfortable having her feet dangle? Stools provide stability.
- Does your child have difficulty communicating when she needs to use the bathroom?
- Is your child sensitive to noise, and does the echo of the bathroom or the flushing of the toilet scare her?
- Does your child have difficulties with body awareness or balance and have difficulty sitting on the toilet seat without support?
- Does your child hold her urine or bowels all day because she is uncomfortable and will not go in the toilet?
- Does your child have a sensitive gag reflex, and the smells in the bathroom are too much to handle?
- Does your child need a visual schedule of what is to be expected when she goes through the "potty" routine?
- Is your child resistant to even trying the potty?

Helpful Tips

- Warm up the toilet seat with a warm towel before using it, and then slowly fade this out.

- Put a stool under your child's feet so she feels secure on the toilet.

- Have the child practice being in the bathroom and getting used to the sounds of people talking, the sink running, and even the toilet flushing before making her use the potty and having to worry about all of that at once.

- Install grab-bars by your toilet for your child to hold on to or help support her physically if she needs it. You can place a pillow behind her and a stool under her feet.

- If your child is afraid of the bathroom, provide her with a safe and comfortable place to use the potty that is *near* the bathroom— maybe put her child-sized potty outside of the bathroom door to start, then gradually move it inside the bathroom.

- Introduce your child to a variety of smells, both pleasant and unpleasant, to help her slowly accommodate to those "not-so-pleasant" smells. Eventually, she will be able to tolerate having a bowel movement in the bathroom. Perhaps you could place a couple of drops of an essential oil on a cotton ball and set it on the countertop.

- Use a visual schedule so she can see the steps involved: Pull pants down, sit on toilet, "pee-pee," wipe, pull pants up, flush, and wash hands. Sometimes having a visual schedule helps.

- Try having a "potty party" with toys and fun things in the bathroom to make it a pleasant and rewarding experience.

Potty Boycott

The first thing you need to do if your child refuses to use the potty outright is to find out what is causing her discomfort. Is it a medical condition? Is she having fears about using the potty? Or fears in other aspects of her life? What is she holding onto? What is she eating? If a child is constipated or has diarrhea, she is not likely to want to potty train. Are you doing the potty training yourself, or is your nanny or daycare provider doing it? Has your child had an experience that has made her uncomfortable in potty training with your nanny or daycare provider? Have you started a dialog with her about what is going on? Is this a battle of wills? Does your child feel that she won't be your special little baby if she's no longer in diapers?

Try to uncover any clues, and if you rule out all of the above, then proceed with potty training in the kindest, firmest, most patient way possible. Let your child know that potty training is not an option, that it is required. She is not going to get to go to kindergarten in pull-ups!

Mistakes Parents Make

- *Forcing a child that is not ready.* If you start potty training and it is a miserable experience for both you and your toddler, try again in a few months, when you have both taken a break and gotten used to the idea that you're going in for round two.

- *Expecting the process to be faster.* It will happen. Some children are super fast, and others take a while to transition to the restroom. Enjoy the journey.

- *Not being understanding about setbacks.* Accidents are going to happen. Sometimes kids get too excited and can't make it to the restroom. Other times they're too tired. Or maybe they just didn't time it right. It's going to take some time to get to 100%. We advise not punishing your little one for having an accident, but saying, "Sometimes this happens, but let's try to go sit on the potty now."

- *Condescending and belittling.* It kills me when parents call their children names or tell them they're acting like a baby or being stupid. If you're trying to get the best out of your child, this is not going to help. All human beings do better when they're encouraged positively.

- *Making a child feel bad about his or her smells.* Do not make your child self-conscious about the way her poop or pee smells. When my son would go potty and the smell bothered him, I used to say,

"Little butt, big smell!" My son thought it was hilarious. I would say, "Now, how did such a little boy make such a big stinky? *That* is impressive." He started telling my husband how he had the stinkiest poops in the world, and he was quite proud of himself.

Britt's Experiences with Potty Training

As my first example of potty training a child with sensory issues, I'll explain the process we used with a little boy with autism, Ethan. I began working with Ethan at the age of 3, when he first received a diagnosis. We struggled through many battles, and one of them was toilet training. In addition to autism, Ethan also had SPD, so his sensory signals weren't organized into appropriate responses. Ethan had difficulty with the way things felt against his skin. He was also sensitive to changes in temperature and had great difficulty wearing certain items of clothing. Most of Ethan's sensitivities were related to his sense of touch, or tactile system.

We made a list of what was and wasn't working for Ethan, including how he did not want to sit on a cold toilet seat. We tried the small child potty, with his favorite characters on it for motivation, but that didn't solve the problem of him wanting to have his bottom close to the water. He preferred to drop his entire little body into the toilet so that his bottom touched the water, perhaps to not make a big splash, or maybe he found the water on his bottom comforting. Ethan wanted to take a bath every time he used the potty, because the sensation felt so awkward to him, that only a bath would calm him and make him feel better. Ethan would sit in his wet underwear until someone realized he was wet and made him go into the bathroom to change. He did not feel the wet sensation against his skin. Because of Ethan's auditory sensitivities, the loud flush of the toilet terrified him.

The next step was to change the environment to help Ethan be successful at using the potty. We warmed the toilet seat with a warm towel before he sat on it, we had the bath ready for him, and we waited until after he left the bathroom to flush the toilet. The biggest step we took was in letting him feel the water with his bottom when he went to the bathroom so he didn't feel like he was falling. We later put a stool under his dangling feet so he felt more secure and grounded. Eventually, with a lot of patience and regular visits to the bathroom, Ethan became potty trained. Keep in mind that Ethan was also receiving sensory-based occupational therapy on a weekly basis to address his many sensory needs, which helped him decrease the tactile defensiveness that he was experiencing.

I would like to share another story of a child that I assisted with using the toilet. This 3-year-old refused to use a traditional bathroom. Her parents and I decided that we could focus on potty training for 2 full days over a weekend. The child was given liquids consistently throughout the 2 days and was taken into the bathroom with toys, books, and videos every 20-30 minutes to sit on the toilet until she was able to urinate. Once she was successful, we threw a party! We danced and played music and gave her a reward. Additionally, the child was allowed to wear as little clothing as possible for her to be comfortable and not restricted by clothes. Every 30 minutes the timer went off, and we took her to the bathroom.

As we moved through the weekend, we increased the time interval between visits to the potty. She continued to drink and eat as much as she wanted throughout the day. We wrapped up simple toys or stickers and let her unwrap them each time she was successful. When we went into the bathroom, we sat there until something happened. Since she was distracted with fun items in the bathroom, it made it easier for her to want to go, and she quickly caught on that if she went potty, then she got a prize and a dance party every time. Within 2 days, she was 90% potty trained and had the confidence to use the toilet with Mom and Dad's assistance. This was a significant turning point in having her stay dry throughout the day, and with Mom and Dad's consistency, she was dry at night within a few weeks.

Staying Dry at Night

While your child is potty-training, you can cover his bed with a protective mattress pad to help keep his mattress dry at night. Or, you could put a water-resistant tablecloth underneath his sheets. I put old towels under the sheets for absorption, just in case.

Sometimes your child will be too tired and will sleep through wetting the bed. Here are some tips to try to help him be successful with staying dry all night:

1. Have him use the potty right before bed.

2. Don't give him any fluids after dinner.

3. Make sure he can pull off his own pajamas when he needs to.

4. Can he see while he's moving from the bed to the bathroom? He may need a night-light.

5. Is he scared of a dark hallway or closet on the way to the bathroom? Again, a night-light may help.

6. Is it too cold for him to get out of bed to go potty? If so, adjust the temperature of your home at night.

7. Try to have him get to the potty early in the morning and then go back to sleep. This way he gets a quick potty trip in, but he's not up for the day yet.

NOTE: Your child's elimination muscles need to be mature enough to hold his urine all night. If these muscles have not developed adequately, he will not physically be able to hold it all night long.

Toddler Hygiene

Haircuts

Some parents choose to cut their baby's hair at home, and some visit a salon. Let's say your child sits nicely with some toys for distraction and has no problem getting his hair cut. Great! Mission accomplished.

Now what if your toddler starts to scream or kick or is unable to sit still? What if he can't be distracted by the movie playing or the silly song you are singing or even for the promise of ice cream if he sits still while you cut? Your child could have sensory issues with auditory sounds or tactile defensiveness or is just plain scared of scissors close to his head, eyes, and ears. What to do? If this seems to be the only area in which your child has trouble, try to make it a pleasant experience for your child. If this seems to be turning into a trend, and he doesn't like having his teeth brushed, his hair washed, his hair cut, or his toenails or fingernails cut, then this might be an issue of tactile defensiveness, and you should seek out an occupational therapy evaluation.

So, what to do? Distract your child—put on a movie, or some of his favorite music. Try giving him a toy, have him sit in your lap, and sing to him or play with him. Don't have him sit in front of a mirror, where he can see the scary sharp things coming at his head—this will only make it worse. Give him headphones to block out the noise. Some parents try to cut their child's hair while he's sleeping, but this can be quite a challenge, as well. Always try to make the situation a positive experience.

Blowing the Nose

Many kids have issues with blowing their noses. Either they don't like having their nose wiped because it's irritating to have Mom squeezing their faces, or the skin is sensitive, and they find it painful. Another problem is that most kids blow out their mouths, not their noses. It takes a while to figure out how to control pushing air out of your nostrils, especially if you're congested or stopped up.

Have your child practice blowing with her mouth first. She can blow whistles, bubbles, pinwheels, flowers, or feathers. Next, try having her take a deep breath in, hold her lips closed, and blow air out her nose. She may need to watch you first and then try it on her own. It is best to master the task of blowing through the nose when the child is not sick, to so that when she is all stuffed up, you can help her get some relief.

Many parents continue to use the suctioning bulb to suction out the goop from their kiddo's nose. Whatever works, right?

Brushing Teeth

Brushing teeth can be a battle for many parents. Trying to hold your child down every night is not a fun way to calm your child down before bed *or* early in the morning, which can lead to starting the day off on the wrong foot. First things first—try various flavors of toothpaste, fun toothbrushes, a vibrating toothbrush, or ones that play music. There's an amazing amount of choices out there. They even have cupcake-flavored dental floss!

Have the child explore the inside of her own mouth with the toothbrush. Then say, "My turn," and you take a turn, even if it's for 2 seconds. Then give control back to the child. Slowly build up to you brushing her teeth, alternating with giving her a turn. Always supervise a child with a toothbrush—you don't want her to fall down and choke with that in their mouth.

MOM TIP: Children either love or hate a vibrating toothbrush, depending on how sensitive their teeth are, but I haven't met a child yet who isn't thrilled to try the musical toothbrushes that play their favorite songs. Let them pick their own toothbrush to promote an interest in brushing.

Nail Trimming

Since your baby was born, you have been clipping his nails. You may have been able to do this while your baby slept blissfully, and now that he's older, you are attempting this activity with your child's participation. Some children are scared of the clippers because they're sharp, they make a clicking sound, and maybe they've had their nails cut too short a few times and it hurts. Other children don't like sitting down through a nail clipping and having their hands or fingers squeezed. Or maybe your toddler already bites his nails.

The reward system may work with this task, or simply talking your child through the process and explaining what you're doing and why you're cutting his nails may suffice. You can be funny, if that works best with your child. Tell him the clippers are eating his nail ends for dessert, yum-yum-yum. Try to clip his nails after a warm bath, when he's relaxed and the nails are softer, or while he's watching his favorite show. Maybe start with his feet first, because it's further away from his eyes, but be careful to not tickle!

You can always continue to cut them while he sleeps if you really have to, but eventually, he should get used to this grooming process.

Bath Time

If you sense that your child is uncomfortable during bath time, maybe fill up the tub before she comes into the bathroom so she doesn't hear the noisy water. Make sure the water temperature is warm, but not too hot. Have toys and maybe bubbles if she likes those things. If she wants to stand in the bathtub because she is uncomfortable sitting, that's okay. Eventually, coax her into a sitting position, even if this takes weeks. Does your child show distress when you tilt her head back to wash her hair? Maybe try placing your hand over her eyes to rinse her hair so she doesn't have to tilt her head back, or have her wear a visor in the bath to keep the water off her face. Even letting your child hold a dry washcloth over her eyes to keep the water out helps.

Does your child show discomfort when you are actually washing her hair? This may be a sign of tactile defensiveness, and if there are other symptoms of tactile defensiveness, then you may want to refer to an occupational therapist in your area to get some help with sensory-processing skills.

Make sure that when it's time to get out of the tub, you have a warm, soft towel to wrap her up in immediately so she doesn't get too cold. A bath mat to stand on is a must, not only to prevent slipping but also to have something soft to stand on instead of the cold tile floor while you are drying her off. Maybe you want to wait to drain the water out of the tub until your child has left the bathroom if she seems to be sensitive to that sort of sound.

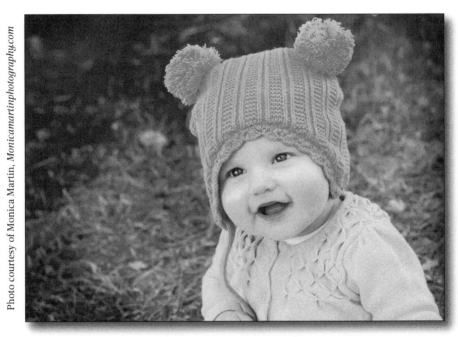

Photo courtesy of Monica Martin, Monicamartinphotography.com

Every day is a new adventure for Payton.
She's ready to take on the world!

Washing Hands

Washing hands is a skill that children will understand and practice more as they get older. At 2 years old, it's impossible to grasp the concept of germs and why we wash our hands so much. The first thing you need to do is make sure that your child can reach the water faucets and is able to turn the water on and off (with supervision, so that he doesn't burn his hands in the hot water). Have him stand on a stool.

It may take a lot of coaxing to get your child to wash his hands, and then once he's there and playing with the bubbles, it's hard to get him to stop! Most importantly, he needs to learn to wash his hands after going to the bathroom and before he eats. If your child really resists washing his hands, use baby wipes to clean his hands sometimes or try a hand sanitizer, although he may reject the consistencies of those items, as well. Try to be patient. Most children will be able to wash their hands appropriately by the time they reach elementary school.

Dressing

Children around 2 years of age should be helping you when you get them dressed. Undressing is much easier, and they may be able to take off their socks and shoes independently. Some toddlers can take off their shirts by themselves or with a little bit of help. They should be able to reach their hands above their heads through the armholes of their shirt and help pull the shirt down over their heads. They will most likely try to pull their pants up at this age, too.

Once you get closer to potty-training time, they should be able to pull their pull-ups down and back up again, or their underwear and pants. Work with your child at this stage to put on his socks and shoes. He should be able to close Velcro fasteners. Children are not usually able to tie their shoelaces properly until around 5 years of age.

Buttons and zippers are hard even for a 4- or 5-year-old child, so don't expect your toddler to be able to button or engage a zipper on a jacket. He could possibly unzip a jacket, though.

Many parents do everything for their child, especially because it's faster, but if you want your child to become more independent, then you should allow him to at least try to do what he can, and then help him along the way. People from different cultures have differing views on how independent toddlers should be, so ask yourself what you would like your toddler to be doing at this point in his life. Would it be easier for him to help dress himself and encourage him to have some autonomy? Or is it easier for you to do it for him?

There are fun dolls available for purchase for both boys and girls that have buttons, zippers, fasteners, and laces for kids to practice on. These are great fine-motor skills to master at any age.

Your Toddler Sleeps

As adults, a siesta is a welcome gift. It's a peaceful time of rejuvenation that we wistfully daydream about, but for toddlers, a nap is a mandatory time-out in their day, during which they could be missing out on exciting adventures! As you most likely know by now, especially if you have older children, it's often difficult for a toddler to switch gears during the day, to drop everything, and to sleep in the afternoon. It helps to start giving your child auditory clues well in advance to start the sleep transition, but, as you know, they will often find any reason they can NOT to sleep. Letting your little one know that after he eats, he is going to get to read two books and then it's nap time, is easier than just sweeping him up off the floor and plopping him in the crib. Be calm but firm with your toddler, and he will learn that when it is naptime, nothing is going to stop it from happening. One long nap a day at this point is sufficient! This is good news for you—you're not as confined to your home as you were before, and both you and your toddler get to enjoy more hours together.

Even though you are more mobile, it is recommended that you go home for naptime. There will always be those magical children that can sleep in the middle of Disneyland, but for the rest of us, being at home in bed is the only way we will doze off. Our brains are incredibly active while we sleep, although scientists are not 100% sure what the brain is working on while we rest. The sleep process is similar to a computer filing and evaluation system—while your toddler sleeps, everything he learns is being processed and filed. New synapses and connections are being generated, and it's possible that anything that is not needed is thrown out. Just think of all the work his body is doing as he grows! If you miss a nap every now and then as your child gets closer to 3 years of age, it is okay, but get him back on a schedule quickly. Naps are still very serious business! You do not want your child falling asleep before dinner and messing up his nighttime sleep schedule. You may need to provide a nap after your toddler comes home from preschool. It is a lot of work to start school!

Where Is Your Toddler Sleeping?

Have you transitioned your toddler from a crib into a toddler bed? Some sleep experts suggest waiting until your toddler is closer to 3 years old. Others recommend using a crib net to keep your climber in the crib a little bit longer. Again, do what works for your family. I loved having my son sleep in my bed and getting to nap while we snuggled.

Have you transformed your baby's room into a toddler room? Did you use all eco-friendly products for your toddler's delicate sensory system? It can be exciting for any child to have a newly decorated room, but make sure it is not overstimulating. If you go with a NASCAR theme, a bright red bed and checkered flags around the room will probably not be calming. It can still be a fun room with a princess bedspread, but remember that the more you have for your toddler to play with and fixate on, the more chances she will be playing in her room instead of sleeping.

Also, now that your child is mobile, how do you know he's going to stay in his bed and not go downstairs and out the doggie door? Make sure that if you do nap while your child naps, your doors are locked and the place is toddler proofed.

Pacifiers: Pros, Cons, Alternatives

Pacifiers are beneficial for sucking and soothing and may help prevent SIDS. Cons include making your child more prone to ear infections and delayed speech development, as well as creating a variety of complications with the teeth protruding forward or the upper and lower jaws not aligning correctly (according to the American Academy of Pediatric Dentistry). Other complications include narrowing of the roof of the mouth.

When it's time to discontinue pacifier use, you can substitute a Chewy Tube, Chewelry (bracelets and necklaces the child can chew on—never leave your child unattended with Chewelry, however), crunchy foods such as pretzels (or gluten-free pretzels), smoothies or milkshakes given through a straw, a popsicle or frozen-juice bar to suck on, use of a vibrating toothbrush in the morning and at night, and toys that have to be blown, such as pinwheels, whistles, and bubbles. For more ideas and information, see *Nobody Ever Told Me (Or My Mother) That! Everything from Bottles and Breathing to Healthy Speech Development,* by Diane Bahr, MS, CCC-SLP.

Pacifiers from an Oral-Motor Perspective

There is an ongoing parenting debate about pacifiers. I, myself, don't have a strong opinion on the subject, as my son never sucked his thumb or used a binky, but many get all heated about the best time to lose the pacifier. Our thoughts are that you should discontinue pacifier use when it is best for you and your child. If your dentist does not see any harm in the pacifier, then is it social pressure? Is it disturbing your child's eating habits? Is it that you don't like looking at it? Or, do you just feel that your child is old enough?

As we have stated in previous chapters, sucking is soothing. Some children need this to calm themselves, and others do not. If you take the pacifier away and your child still craves that oral-motor suck, let her drink a milkshake or smoothie through a straw with your supervision, in the morning and afternoon (if you let her have one at night, she may have to go to the bathroom). Many children give their pacifier up easily after having transitioned to only having it at night for a few months. Parenting can be easier than we think when we are a little bit more relaxed about it. Some experts say that the binky should be phased out around 18 to 24 months. Some families even use the balloon method, where you tie the binky to the balloon and give it a "good-bye party." If your child has special needs or still needs help calming and soothing himself, you may need to use the binky for even longer than 24 months, which is okay. You need to decide what's best for you and your family.

Good Night, Toddler!

After a busy day, your toddler may often be eager for bed, but not if it becomes Wrestle Mania time with Daddy! I get so frustrated when my husband comes in during the bedtime routine, and before I know it, my son is hanging off of his back and jumping off the bed. It can take a good hour to calm him back down after all that excitement. Talk to your partner and your older children about not getting your toddler riled up before bed. It's not fair to you or to your child. Your dog and your neighbors can be culprits, too. Whip out your Sleep Police badge and keep everyone calm during bedtime.

Un-oh! Are you on the overtired toddler train? We know how hard it can be to get your toddler back into a positive sleep cycle once your little one is overly exhausted. If your toddler is not getting a good amount of sleep or deep enough sleep during his nap, it makes it harder the next time he goes to bed. This is another reason the sleeping schedule is so important. You have to stick to it as long as you can.

Let the Sunshine in!

If your toddler is slow to rise in the morning, help her out by letting the sunshine in. Our bodies naturally adjust to being awake if we see sunlight. Open the drapes, the shutters, or the blinds. Who cares what the neighbors think of you in your pajamas?

Social Skills

Many are often surprised to find social skills addressed by occupational therapists; however, how could you have an occupation without social skills? Your toddler is going to learn most of her social skills from you and the rest of your family, until she enters the world of school and learns all kinds of negative behaviors you'll get to work on. Sigh. But for now, your toddler will mirror how you greet people, how you interact with others, and how you socialize. If you say "Hello, glad to meet you," upon meeting a new person, chances are your child will learn this skill. Some kids are more observant than others, and some will need more instruction on how to be a good friend.

Start with the basics. Make sure you show your child the proper way to greet people and to say good-bye. Some parents encourage their kids to hug and kiss everyone—that's your choice. Others keep it simple with a handshake or a wave hello and good-bye. You may also start introducing manners at this time. "Please" and "thank you" are "magic" words that your toddler will only learn if you use them yourself.

As your toddler grows, it's important that she is able to function and communicate with others. This is your responsibility. If your child is tucked away in your home until she starts kindergarten, chances are she's not going to be able to function within a social environment. If your child has developmental delays or special needs, she may need social-skills classes to assist her in a social environment. Britt has taught various social-skills classes that have been very successful for children. Some of them have included pairing children with fewer social skills with other children who have strong social skills and having them play and interact together, participating in games like hide-and-seek and teamwork games like "Mother May I?" and "Red Rover." Some of these are geared toward older children, as you can see, but you get the idea of how to get children to interact. One child was never very good at being "found" during hide-and-seek and would cry and become very upset with his peers. With some coaching and practice, he was finally able to play this game with his friends. For younger children, giving them the foundation for developing social skills can help prevent more difficult times down the road, but let's face it—at some point in our lives, we have ALL been socially awkward (especially in middle school—YIKES!).

Jackie's son is currently in a social-skills class, as well as a "Think it through" class, because he doesn't quite understand behaviors and the choices kids are making in school. He's currently working on how to join a group at recess and how to find appropriate topics to discuss with friends. During toddler social-skills class, your child will learn about things like boundaries. My son learned to tell people to stop when they got to close to him. It's about arming the child with verbal and physical cues if he's not picking them up naturally.

I've noticed that children who are not taught how to interact properly with others have difficulty in school and in social environments, which is going to lead to difficulties when they enter the work force.

Start now parents, NOW.

If your child is in daycare or any other structured classes, find out from the caretakers and instructors what type of social skills they work on during the day. Most will teach the rules of respecting each other, sharing, taking turns, winning and losing, and not always getting picked for every activity.

Playdates

The world of playdates is an interesting beast. Some people prefer one-on-one playdates, while others choose a large group. There are free playdates that parents organize, and there are pay playdates through organizations. All are good for toddlers. The key is to find a playgroup for your lifestyle. Do you prefer weekend playdates, involving activities in the park or at the zoo? Do you enjoy hosting playdates and providing a neutral environment? Have you checked with your religious affiliation for playdate arrangements? There are many to choose from, so find a group that works for your family. There are many playgroups posted online for your convenience.

Playdate Rules

Some playdates may be relaxed, and the parents chat instead of enforcing rules and providing guidance to the toddlers. Do not hesitate in leaving a group if one child is always kicking, hitting, or biting and his parent does nothing to correct this behavior. It's up to you to make sure your toddler is safe and doesn't learn those habits. If your child is the kicker, hitter, or biter, then it is YOUR responsibility to redirect your toddler and stop her before she can harm another child. Also, find out why your child is doing this. Are you a hitter, kicker, or biter? Has she learned this from you or your partner? Does she have siblings that are forceful with her, and she's learned how to fight as a reflex? Is she frustrated that she can't get her way with another child and doesn't know how to ask for it? Is she uncomfortable in social environments? Does she have communication delays?

Your Role

There is a balance between hovering over your child during a playdate and completely leaving her to fend for herself. No child is going to want her mother in her face, correcting her every move while she plays, but then your child will also look to you for guidance if her play-date buddy dumps a cup of juice on her head. You are responsible for your child's safety during a playdate. If she's jumping on the couch, physically remove her from the couch. If she's pulling a dog's tail, remove her hand from the dog. If your child is playing or parallel-playing with another child and they're doing just fine, sit back and enjoy a cup of tea and chat with the other moms. Enjoy this time. Exchange recipes and talk about the best local outings they've experienced.

Worry Wart

Like we've said before, your child will mirror you. It will be hard for your toddler to relax and stay calm in the playdate environment if you're on edge, panicking about every detail. Whether you're right next to your child or not, she will feel your manic energy and be nervous herself. Try to keep yourself calm, even if you are intimidated by the other moms or are anxious that the playdate will not go well. Controlling your internal system always aids your toddler in controlling hers.

Sharing

Like all parents, we dream of our children being philanthropic, giving the shirt off their backs to a homeless child you pass on the street. Most likely, however, your toddler will not want to share, so these dreams will have to wait until your child is old enough to learn about being empathetic toward others. Sharing is a skill that your toddler needs to learn, primarily in a social environment or at home if he has siblings, yet we also understand how a child does not always want to share. My husband still won't share, and he's in his 30s! His toys are his toys. And is this really a bad thing? What we suggest is that your child has a des-ignated special toy that he doesn't have to share and could put away before company arrives for a playdate. This will make sharing all the rest of his toys that much easier. It's natural for your toddler to want to keep some things private and special, so having a healthy compromise will create a more peaceful playdate when your guests dive head-first into your toddler's toy box.

What Ifs

What if my toddler has no interest in other kids whatsoever? What if my toddler hides and barks if taken to a social class? What if my child experiences sheer terror of others at the park and won't get out of his stroller? What if my child is violent toward other kids on playdates? If you find that your child has extreme social aversions, please take him to your pediatrician and get a referral to an occupational therapist for an evaluation. This is not something your child will just grow out of on his own by forcing him to go onto the playground or in the classroom or participate in any other activity without professional help. Britt helps parents with these types of concerns every day. An occupational therapist can evaluate your child to see if this is caused by SPD or a social-anxiety disorder. A developmental psychologist would be able to help, as well.

Tantrums, Discipline, Redirecting, and Prevention

Tantrums

If you study how our brains mature, you can take a little bit of the guesswork out of tantrums. Research has shown that a child's brain does not develop symbolic reasoning and understanding (the ability to think about things in more than one way and then understand how the world operates) until he is nearly 3 years old. This means that if you're asking your child to perform certain tasks that require brain functions he has not yet developed, then you are pretty much asking for a tantrum. John Medina, of *Brain Rules,* says, "We don't appear to do much to distinguish ourselves from apes before we are out of the terrible twos."[8]

When you understand your toddler's brain's capacity, you can adjust your expectations accordingly. We will try to help you deal with a toddler's full-blown eruption—because it's going to happen. No one gets through parenting without tantrums. The first thing parents need to do is make sure their little Tasmanian devil is safe from harm and from themselves. Do not let her bang her head on the tile floor or lay in the street where there's traffic. Protect your toddler during her blast of emotion.

- *The "I want it now!" tantrum.* This most common tantrum can hit at any moment. Whether it is a toy, or food, or an item that an older sibling has, when a toddler wants something, she wants it immediately—and she will SPAZ out if she doesn't get it. The worst thing you can do is to give her the desired item during a full-blown tantrum. If you planned on giving her the toy or item, tell her that she may have the toy, but not until she's completely calm. Wait for the tantrum to pass, and then give her the desired item. Do not reward negative behavior by giving in to the child mid-tantrum.

- *The "I don't want to do that" tantrum.* I don't want to wear that shirt, I don't want to eat that food, I don't want to leave the sandbox! These tantrums result from your toddler expressing her independence and her desires in an unattractive and usually noisy blast of emotion that travels through her body. As with the previous type of tantrum, let it pass, and then either give your child a choice or another warning that she will be leaving the sandbox shortly, tantrum or not.

- *The "I don't know what I want" tantrum.* Okay, admit it, we all have days when everything just feels off, and we aren't thinking clearly. These tantrums can come out of nowhere and pass without any explanation. Your toddler might be hungry, tired, or irritated; her sensory system might be agitated; she might have a cold coming on; it could be anything. We know, a lot of help that is! But sometimes, being understanding and knowing that your toddler is doing her best to get through what she's feeling can be enough. Let the tantrum pass, see if you can find a lesson for your child in it, and move on. Never hold a grudge against your child for throwing a tantrum, even if she has thrown herself down in the middle of your favorite restaurant in front of your high-school friends, whom you have not seen in 20 years. Get over it. It happens to all of us.

Discipline

When your child misbehaves, it can be easy for your blood to go from 98.6° to boiling in one heartbeat. As a parent, you may have to practice stepping back and calming yourself down before you can discipline your child. I, personally, have had to step aside and ask my husband to take over, and he has done the same. If I am too heated to discipline safely and effectively, then I give myself a time-out. If no one is there to relieve me in my time of stress, I have told my son that "Mommy needs a minute," and made sure he was safely in his room or playpen while I practiced some deep breathing. We're human—at times we're going to blow up, get angry, and feel defeated. It is how we *deal* with our own emotions that sets an example for our children.

I've read that 50% of parents spank their kids. I was a child who was spanked, and yes, I am a functioning adult and don't hate my parents, but I do not hit my child, and I do not recommended it for any situation. I do not believe it is effective. Hitting does not teach a child anything meaningful, but it *does* promote fear and violence and break down communication. Parents often feel guilty after spanking their children and they might give them something to make them feel better, which teaches a child to play on their parents' guilt. Basically, there just isn't anything positive that comes out of hitting a child.

Is There an Echo in Here?

One thing parents need to be aware of when disciplining, however they choose to do so, is to not discipline a child for mirroring the parents' own behavior. Our little ones learn from watching us, and they mimic our words, our actions and behaviors, and our mannerisms, and they use our phrases and dialect. As we've stated before, our children can be reflections of us at times, matching their sensory systems and emotions to ours. If you're constantly scolding the dog, chances are you will hear your toddler scold the dog the same way. If you talk negatively to your toddler, I can almost guarantee she will talk negatively back to you. It is human nature, and it is what a child has been taught. Before disciplining, perhaps you should check yourself and see if it is your own behavior that needs to be modified.

Toddlers who attend daycare or playdates in the park or have older siblings will learn a lot of negative behaviors and phrases and will try them out on you for a reaction. At times it can be shocking and at other times humorous when they use phrases out of context—but, again, remember to use these times to teach your child what is acceptable behavior and what is not.

Time-Outs

Many parents find time-outs effective when their children are really young. If you'd like visual demonstrations of how to implement a kind and firm time-out, watch ABC's "Supernanny," featuring Jo Frost. She's the perfect example of how kids respond to her authoritative presence. She's never mean or cruel and is always consistent and unwavering.

Recently, I attended a conference on behaviors, and many of the experts are saying to increase the amount of one-on-one time you spend with your child and give him LOTS of positive praise so that when he does something that is not "okay" (ie, throwing a toy, hitting, biting, spitting, or throwing himself on the floor), you do not accidentally reinforce the negative behavior by giving it too much attention. You just simply say, "That behavior is not okay," and pick him up and put him in a time-out chair or a specific place designated for "time-outs." Research suggests that you should have the child sit for the minute equivalent of his age (ie, if he's 2 years old, have him sit for 2 minutes), and then when he comes out of "time-out," he has to either clean up the toy he threw or apologize to whomever he hit, etcetera.

Parenting with Love and Logic

One approach that I suggest to families that I work with is called "Parenting with Love and Logic," created by Jim Fay *(www.loveandlogic.com).* Jim and his son Charles and many other trained speakers travel all over the country giving presentations about how to parent with love and logic in mind. My favorite tool to use especially with young children, between 2 and 5 years of age, is "Bummer, Mark, I am so sorry that you are not able to have a lollypop right now. You have to eat your dinner first. Yes, I understand that you are frustrated, and you can cry if you like, but we are not eating candy before dinner." This would be spoken in a calm, regulatory voice, never getting mad or upset that the child is throwing a HUGE tantrum in the middle of Target.

Another example might be when your 2-year-old continues to pull objects out from underneath your bathroom sink and scatters them all over the floor. You calmly approach your child and tell her, "Kelly, you cannot pull out Mommy's stuff from the cabinets." Then you pick her up, move her into another room, and provide a different form of entertainment for her. She may throw herself on the floor, try to run back into the bathroom, or just scream really loudly. Your blood may boil, as you are exhausted from working all day, cooking dinner, cleaning up the house, and doing laundry, but you are going to STOP and take five deep breaths, and not let your toddler know that she is getting to you. Remember, YOU are the parent, YOU are in charge, and your little toddler has to follow the rules of the house.

There are many ways to parent your child, and we are not here to tell you which one is right and which one is wrong, but I can tell you from watching many families interact and watching many parents discipline (or NOT discipline) their children, the one thing that seems to make everyone upset is when the parent or caregiver raises his or her voice and yells at the child. I understand this is hard not to do when you've just "had it"! But I encourage you to find your inner self and relax and realize that in the scheme of things, Johnny wanting a lollypop and throwing a tantrum in the middle of Target is not the end of the world. If you need to scream or yell, do it in your bedroom with the door closed. Don't do it in front of your child. Trying to reason with a toddler or a young child who is already upset is not going to get you anywhere.

Applied Behavioral Analysis

Applied Behavioral Analysis, or ABA, is widely used in the treatment of children with autism. As an experienced ABA therapist prior to becoming an occupational therapist, I believe that some of the basic components of this approach work with typically developing children as well as children with special needs. Most children, if not all children, will have problems with their behaviors at some time. The ABA model supports positive reinforcement for children to learn a new skill or task. When you are trying to teach a child a new skill, sometimes he just learns it because he is intrinsically inspired to learn something new, and verbal praise is enough for him to want to please you. For some children, this is not the case. Many times, you have to repeatedly show a child the same thing over and over again and maybe even physically help him complete the task. Take stacking blocks as an example. Maybe your child is 2 already, and he is unable to stack even two small blocks. You can show him, help him physically, and when he does it (even if you helped him), praise him, clap for him, and reward him for completing the task. Then repeat the task again so he can learn the motor-memory pattern of how to stack the block on top of the other one. Don't punish him if he knocks it over, just help him try again. You will find that there are some things that your child excels in and other things are more difficult to conquer. This is typical, and you shouldn't be worried if your child struggles here or there with a fcw things that maybc another child in your Mommy & Me class is doing really well.

Redirecting, Redirecting, Redirecting

I learned how to implement redirecting my son by watching Britt work with him. I can honestly say she taught me how to be a better parent without realizing it. Observing the way she didn't constantly say, "No, don't do that. No. No," as I often heard myself doing, was refreshing.

What she *would* do was redirect him away from the behavior she didn't approve of. If he was putting his hands down his pants, she's say, "Let's put our hands on the table." See how she didn't acknowledge his hands down his pants, yell at him, or say 'no'? She would redirect him, and, through showing him what was acceptable, he learned and didn't get scolded, and I didn't get upset. It was a pleasant change.

I also learned that I had to redirect often. It got to be days and days of redirecting, but there were fewer meltdowns and power struggles, and his tantrums disappeared. I also find that this works with husbands!

Prevention

The most important thing you can do is to set your child up for developmental and sensory success. If you don't want to have to constantly discipline your child at home, make your home a safe haven, where your child won't be tempted to play with Mommy's Beanie Baby collection. Don't leave cookies on the counter and then tell your child he can't have them. Outside the home, don't take him to the park hungry and then not expect a tantrum. There are many times when a child is reacting to you or a situation that could have been avoided. Take responsibility for these times and be more prepared the next time. I, for one, am constantly learning new ways to be a better parent, and I'm learning to think ahead. I'm always trading new information with fellow parents. You mean I *shouldn't* have expected my child to be able to run ten errands with me and THEN attend dinner with my husband's boss's family? Sometimes my expectations are just unrealistic.

You may say, "Well that's just life." You are right, but for the sake of your sanity and that of your child, not to mention your relationship, why not make your days as smooth as possible and save the discipline for necessary learning experiences? Yelling at your child for wanting a cookie isn't teaching him anything or preparing him to be a functional and fulfilled adult.

Outings

I constantly have other parents telling me, "Well, it was fine when *we* were kids." Yes, yes, I get it. Kids are resilient, and we all turned out fine after riding in the back of the station wagon with no seat belts, getting vaccinations and spankings, and wearing wet swimsuits home from the beach. I hear you. Yes, I know your mothers drank and smoked while pregnant, and you're "fine." It's also a bit different now, because the world is moving at a faster pace than it was then. People work longer hours, get more done in a day than they used to in a week, and are able to communicate with every corner of the world with the touch of a button. We come into contact with more toxins than ever before, and we're a sicker country than ever before, so maybe, just maybe, we're not all as "fine" as we think. It can only help to be considerate of your toddler's sensory needs, and why not even be considerate of your own? Both you and your toddler will feel better, and by doing so, you'll be creating a more peaceful and healthy lifestyle.

Clothing is a big issue during outings. If you plan to have your toddler out all day, bring a sweater or coat for the evening. Bring dry clothes if you may get wet (or in case of accidents) and keep spare undergarments in the car, just in case.

Do not leave home without SNACKS. If your child's blood sugar is low or she gets hungry, you are guaranteed to have a meltdown. Avoid this by providing her with healthy snacks and keep your toddler hydrated.

Now, off to your adventures!

Arcades

If you have older children, or your partner behaves like a big child (hey, it can be fun, we're not knocking it), then chances are you'll find yourself at an arcade of some sort, whether it be a Chuck E. Cheese, Dave & Buster's, or a carnival or fair type of setting. Games are all the rage, and even though there are Wiis and an X-box in almost every household, people still like to get out and play games they don't own. While this may be exciting and fun for a toddler, after a short amount of time, this could be overstimulating and lead to a meltdown. The sounds of the games, people yelling or cheering, and music pumping can be a lot to take in. There is also lots of candy, sodas, and junk food at those places, which will add to a toddler's system being off-kilter. Enjoy your time there, but watch for an overstimulated child who is trying to drown out the commotion, or take note if your child is getting too aggressive and cranky. If your older kids don't want to leave, maybe take a sensory break with your toddler, walk around the outside of the arcade, and look at flowers or rocks. Let your toddler collect herself before taking on another game of Whack-the-Gopher.

The Beach

A day at the beach can start as a magical adventure—wind blowing, waves crashing, sand in your toddler's toes. After a few hours of the

sun beating down on you, finding sand in your sandwich, and salty water burning a cut on your toddler's foot, however, life isn't as fabulous. Make sure you plan your time at the beach around snacks and naps, and *always* bring dry clothes for your toddler to change into after you've wiped sand off a few times at the car. Some beaches have a shower area to wash off the sand. It may be worth the few moments in cold water to get your toddler cleaned up before a long car ride.

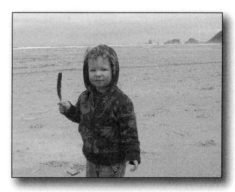

Asher the adventurer enjoying the beach and the simple joys of a feather.
ASHER, 2 YEARS OLD

If you frequent the beach, your toddler will most likely adapt to a day of sun, sand, wind, and salty water, but for those of you who make the beach a once-a-year outing, don't force a year's worth of fun into one day. You can only make so many sandcastles and search for so many shells before your toddler is going to burn out and need to go inside. If you're staying at a hotel on a beach, give your toddler some quiet time in the hotel room to cool down and regulate herself before heading off on a whale-watching excursion.

Make sure to reapply sunscreen often, as a sunburn is sure to have negative results on your toddler's skin and sensory systems.

MOM TIP: If your toddler runs at the sight of your tube of sunscreen and you've tried the sprays, lotions, and colorful zinc oxides, then try UPF 50+ clothing, available at numerous stores online, such as www.coolibar.com. It's not only rash guards. They are stocked with colorful, stylish hoodies, active-wear shirts, and the all-important HATS, in addition to swimwear for babies and toddlers. They're great for the beach or any outdoor adventure! Be sure to use sunscreen on your child's face, hands, and feet if they're exposed.

Church

Fortunately, most places of worship have an area for children, and they are also open and loving toward children. If you would like to bring your baby or your toddler into your place of worship, then think about what is best for you and the congregation. Do you need to have a few toys for your toddler to play with? Will you be too distracted with taking care of your toddler to focus? Remember that is it hard for a little one to sit for an hour with nothing to occupy her attention, and toddlers need to move their bodies.

Dentists and Doctors

A trip to the doctor can be an adventure. There are different smells in the waiting room, as well as new noises, and it can be scary for a doctor or dentist to poke and examine you. If your dentist and/or doctor's waiting room does not have activities for kids, bring your own to help your toddler calm himself down before going in to see the doctor. Coloring or stringing beads can be a soothing activity while waiting. Don't bring LeapFrog games or a DS, as those are stimulating, and your toddler might become upset if he has to stop playing when he's called in.

If your child shows anxiety about having a check-up, go to the library and get books on the topic to read with him. Talk to him about what doctors and dentists do and how they help keep you healthy and strong. Get a pretend doctor's kit, and let your toddler go through the motions of checking your temperature and blood pressure and looking in your ears. Also, bring along your toddler's comfort item, like a stuffed animal or blanket.

Try to stay calm inside the room while the doctor and nurses examine your child. Our children feed off of our energy, and if we're nervous or anxious, then they get nervous and anxious too. Don't have unreasonably high expectations of your child in the dentist's or doctor's office. If he's scared, comfort him and encourage him to try and open his mouth. Yelling at him or forcing him is not going to make the experience any better for him, you, or your doctor, and then the next trip will be even worse. It's better to start a reward system. If your toddler opens his mouth wide for the dentist, then he'll get a sticker or get to watch his favorite movie before bed. Some parents will purchase an item for their child as a reward if the doctor's appointment has been particularly stressful (such as shots or stitches), but that is on a per-parent basis.

Farmers' Markets

An outdoor market can be a lot of fun for families to explore together. It's good for your toddler to see the fresh fruits and vegetables and get to pick ones she would like to try. Some farmers' markets have horse rides and other forms of outdoor entertainment. Be aware if your toddler is getting overstimulated. Is her nose running from the horses' hay? Is the live music too loud, and is your child trying to drown it out? Is it getting cold out, and you forgot a jacket? If your toddler is doing well, enjoy a few hours, have a picnic, and dance on a grassy lawn, but if your toddler has had enough, go home or take a walk away from the hubbub to give her some time to regulate.

Grocery Store

The grocery store can be a torture chamber for both toddlers and parents. A visit to the grocery store often starts on a bad foot because we're hungry and in a hurry. These two things make us cranky and can spell trouble for our toddler, too. There are a few things to consider that might be causing you and your toddler additional discomfort. The lights in the grocery store are often fluorescent and can cause a headache. The grocery carts are hard and cold, uncomfortable for your toddler to sit in, and infested with germs. Often there is music playing in the grocery store, which can make it hard to focus, and aisles and aisles of food, which your toddler may or may not find interesting.

How can you make your trip to the grocery store more enjoyable? Have a list! Know what you're there to get and ask your toddler to help you find the items. Have a plan. Start at one end of the store and finish at the opposite end. Going back and forth to different aisles won't save time, and you may forget items you need.

Bring sunglasses for your toddler if the lights in the grocery store bother her eyes. Bring a book with musical buttons for your toddler to push every time you put an item in the cart. Act silly! Walk like different animals while you push the cart, flap your arms like a chicken, swing your arm like an elephant trunk. Your toddler (not to mention your fellow shoppers) will be thrilled at your ability to be goofy in public and will be far too entertained to throw a tantrum.

Always reward good behavior in the grocery store to make your trips more pleasant. If you're going to let your toddler pick out a cereal, a popsicle treat, or some special crackers, talk about it as you enter the store. Say, "Olivia, have you decided what special crackers you'd like to get?" Make going to the grocery store an opportunity to develop a healthy relationship with food. Ask your toddler, "Does lettuce grow in the ground or from a tree?" "Do you think monkeys would like these bananas as much as Daddy?" Or better yet, have Daddy or your partner take over grocery duty with your toddler every now and then. Ask your toddler to let Daddy know how the trip to the grocery store works. Some toddlers love authority.

Library

Local libraries often have a story time for young children. Sometimes they might do puppet shows along with the books, but usually, a librarian reads up at the front of the room. Some kids love to listen to books being read aloud and eagerly await the pictures of the book, but others find it hard to sit through a story when they're very young. My son was far more interested in the computers at the library and looking through the books himself than sitting and listening in story time. We don't recommend forcing your child to sit still for a story if he's not ready yet. You might prepare him beforehand with a walk or jumping jacks to get out some of his energy. It may take a while for your child to learn to regulate his inside voice, and a library is a great place to practice. Most librarians are as fond of children as they are books and will help teach your child the rules of the library.

The Mall

Once your child is a teenager, the mall will most likely become her home away from home, but as a toddler, the mall can be a sensory challenge. The lighting is, again, often fluorescent. There is usually loud music pumping in the main areas of the shopping center, as well as different music blaring in some of the stores. Stores like Abercrombie & Fitch have even taken the lights down low, making it dark in addition to loud. It feels more like a nightclub than a clothing store. These sudden sensory changes can be challenging to an adult, let alone a toddler. Give her time to adjust to each store and environment and be ready to leave the mall if your child is tired or hungry. Another option is to plan a time for your toddler to play in a mall playground area or to see the puppies at the pet store if she's been patient, while Mommy tries on clothes in JCPenny for half an hour.

Movies

Some parents choose to take their babies and toddlers to the movies. Please note that just because your child may be able to sleep through "Slasher Fest 4," this movie choice is not good for your baby's brain development and sensory system. If your baby cries during "Sleepless in Seattle 2," it is courteous to take your baby into the lobby, for both the audience's sake and that of your baby and/or toddler. If your child cries during a movie, he may be suffering from an auditory issue or the lights being down, the movie lights flashing, and the loud music and sounds. It may just be complete sensory overload.

Children's movies are more appropriate for your child, and the audience is more flexible with regard to your child's outbursts, laughing, talking, and crying. If your child has sound sensitivities, check with your theater about quieter showings or find out if they have a quiet box for children with autism and sensory-processing issues. This is becoming more and more popular at theaters nationwide.

Museums (for Kids)

Discovery museums for kids are FUN! Don't try and take your toddler to see the Mona Lisa. A 2-year-old is not going to appreciate the art of being carted through a quiet museum for an afternoon, unless he's asleep in a stroller. Also, those that are there to actually appreciate the art exhibit will not appreciate you bringing in a noisy toddler during their art experience. While we don't often say that a mother should alter her life for others just because she has kids, museums are one of the areas where it's just not okay to ask other adults to accommodate your child, especially since there are children's museums that are educational and exciting for your toddler. If you insist on taking your toddler to a museum exhibit, make sure to bring a book or a quiet toy for your child to play with while you get a closer look at that Van Gogh.

Park

Parks are the romping ground of toddlers. This is where they can explore, play, climb, be free, and socialize. What they don't know is that they're working all their sensory systems. They're using their motor skills while climbing, their vestibular sense while swinging, their tactile sense while sifting sand, and their auditory sense while listening to the other kids and the birds chirping. They're also processing countless amounts of sensory input. At times the park can be peaceful, and at other times, overwhelming. There are a lot of social rules at the park, and it can be a place in which to create positive social skills, such as sharing a shovel brought from home, or taking turns on the slide. The park is also a lot of work for Mommy or Daddy if they use the park to guide their toddler's behaviors instead of sitting on a bench reading the latest John Grisham novel while their child throws sand in another toddler's eyes.

Without hovering too much, help your child engage with the other children at the park. You may also talk to the other parents and nannies, which will exemplify for your child the way polite introductions and conversation are made. Use other children's poor behavior as a teaching tool, too. You can say, "We don't throw sand at others." Or, help your child learn to wait for his turn on the slide. "Almost your turn, Joey. Only two more kids ahead of you. Good waiting!"

Again, watch your child for cues. If he's tired or overstimulated, cut your trip to the park short. Also, if the older kids there are being too aggressive, don't wait for your toddler to get trampled before getting him out of harm's way.

If it is summertime and your park has a water-spray area for the kids to play in, then bring an extra outfit for your toddler to change into. Carting around a wet child isn't fun for you or him.

Restaurants

While restaurants can be enjoyable for adults to sit and dine for hours, it's not as fun for a toddler, unless you're at Chuck E. Cheese. If the restaurant is not kid friendly, bring your own coloring books and crayons, as well as a variety of other toys if you're going to be there for an extended period of time. It's not natural for a child to sit at a table for 2 hours at such a young age, so she will probably need for you or your partner to take her on a walk around the building to get some energy out. Britt and I created a spandex and nylon Play Pouch for parents to use in restaurants, as well as while traveling. The fabric is as strong as rubber, giving your child a workout while seated at the table, while you have more time to chat with your friends and family. For more information, visit our Web site at *www.sensoryparenting.com.*

If you take your child to a fast-food restaurant with a playground inside, make sure you establish the rules of playing before you get there. The child should eat first and then play. Also, follow the rules of the playground by removing your shoes if you are instructed to. Be careful if your child spooks easily around other children. My son crawled up into a tube at McDonalds and then screamed for dear life when another child came up the tube. It was difficult to climb up there myself and get him out, and it took a long time to calm him down afterward. Pick a time when it's not crowded to let your child get comfortable with the equipment.

Theme Parks

Perhaps you have dreamed of the day when you could introduce your little angel to the princesses of Disney, and now that day has arrived. Or maybe your nephew's having his third birthday party at Camp Snoopy, and you have to attend or your sister will be upset. Either way, here is some "been there, done that" advice on embracing a theme park with your toddler.

Bring a stroller or rent one. A toddler can only walk so much before exhaustion will kick in. Save yourself from having to chase your little man through a crowd. You will also have storage for the trinkets you accumulate and a place to put your hot chocolate down during the electric light–show parade.

MOM TIP: Always have an exit strategy. If your toddler is super sensitive to sound and you're going to sit through an hour of "Snow White" in an outdoor amphitheater, then sit by an aisle where you can take your child and leave if he has a total meltdown. Also, be mindful of speaker placement. Don't sit next to a speaker bigger than your body that will be pumping "High Ho" at unthinkable decibels. And if you sit in the front row at a whale show at Seaworld, you are going to get wet—so keep your extra set of clothes dry!

Your toddler is going to need to nap at some point during a long theme park day, and the issue is that there are not any quiet places to sneak away to for the auditory-sensitive child. If you don't have a hotel to escape to, then insist on a "rest" stroll, with your child snuggled up in the stroller. Find a boring section of the park and pace back and forth until your child falls asleep. It may take a while for him to give in to the sleep fairies, but it will be worth it if you plan on staying late to see the fireworks.

Do not skip meals, and don't get suckered into purchasing a lifetime supply of cotton candy. Most theme parks have fruit and healthier food options scattered through the park; however, they may charge nine dollars for a banana. Think ahead, pack your own lunch, and eat at the designated picnic areas.

AUTISM MOM TIP: If you are worried about going to Disneyland because your child has autism, go to their guest services desk at City Hall and inquire about their disability passes (which are similar to a "Fast Pass"). You and your child will not have to wait in the long lines in the park, which can be far too much on your child's sensory system and your sanity. You may have to show proof of your child's diagnosis on a doctor's letterhead. Call BEFORE going to the park so that you're aware of the current requirements to get this pass. If you plan your trip well in advance, request a "Guidebook for Guests with Disabilities."

Not all children enjoy rides, particularly those that are prone to car and or/motion sickness. Rides are extreme exercise for all of your sensory systems. They're usually blaring some sort of music throughout the ride, and your vision is working with your vestibular system so that you can see clearly while being catapulted through the sky. While some kids love rides and will beg to go on Mr Toad's Wild Ride repeatedly through the day, others will squirm and throw a tantrum after waiting in line for an hour. If your child's anxiety peaks before a ride, be willing to walk away and try taking him on the ride at another time.

There's safety in numbers! You don't want to back yourself into a corner by being the only adult with more than one child in line for a ride. Most rides are for two people to sit by one another, so unless you take a seat by yourself, one kid may be left alone on the ride. Bring a friend or your partner and save yourself from the headache of wrestling two boys into the handicapped bathroom stall while you try to pee. This will also help you and the child who does want to go on a ride if you have to take the emergency exit at the front of the ride with your screaming toddler.

Travel

With any motion, there is a possibility that motion sickness will ensue. This occurs when all the messages to the brain from the skin, eyes, and ears are saying one thing, and the brain is not processing the information, which causes nausea and sickness. You'll know early on if your child is prone to motion sickness and learn tools to help ease and avoid the symptoms. Encourage your toddler to face forward and look outside. Don't let her read (if she can) or play a travel game that will worsen her symptoms. Avoid placing the child prone to motion sickness in the very back seat of the minivan and be ready to open the window for a bit if your child needs some fresh air to help ease the queasiness. Talk to your doctor before trying any medicines or any homeopathic remedies.

Road trips are fantastic family adventures, but you must be well prepared for your trip to run smoothly. Whether you're traveling by car, plane, or train, you must have a bag full of activities and snacks for your toddler. For road trips, a lot of cars are equipped with DVD players and game outlets. While you may use those from time to time, don't forget the classic games, like counting all the red cars that go by or singing as a family. Find stops on your route that will be entertaining and educational. Is the world's largest ball of string at an exit mid-trip? What about a reptile house? These stops can break up a monotonous car ride and sometimes end up being the coolest part of your trip.

Taking a toddler through airport security can be a challenge. Especially if you have a baby, too! Nowadays, you have to take your baby out of her carrier, take off everyone's shoes and jackets, and wait in line—sometimes for HOURS. This is hard on you as a parent and is extremely difficult for your toddler. This is when snacks and activities come in handy. Don't worry about other passengers being annoyed and just try to keep you and your toddler on track. It can be frightening for your child to walk through a security metal detector alone with a big man standing there observing her with a paddle device in his hands. Talk to your toddler and explain that they're looking for metal objects like when Grandpa Joe tried to find treasure at the beach with his funny device.

Once you are on the tarmac, have more activities planned for your toddler. A good idea would be to get a bag of new items that your child hasn't already played with to keep her occupied for a long flight. You can also try our Play Pouch, which helps your child let out her energy constructively while in her seat. Try to keep your child from turning around and bothering passengers behind you and—most of all—try and keep her from kicking the seat in front of her. Remember, we practice being considerate to our sensory systems, as well as to strangers on a plane. To prevent your child's ears from popping while landing, encourage her to have a snack or sip on water to promote swallowing while the airplane descends.

The train is an exciting adventure, until your child gets motion sickness. Trains move fast and stop suddenly, so your toddler will need to hold onto you or a railing if you're standing up while the train is moving. If your child gets motion sickness on a train, hold her in your lap and have her sip water until the train stops. Bring along peppermints or ginger-root capsules, both of which are known to calm a queasy stomach.

Some children love to be out at sea, while others can't stomach it. Perhaps you should go on a short boat ride (either fishing or a tour) to see if your child gets seasick before booking a week-long Nickelodeon Sea Adventure with Spongebob. If you do find yourself out at sea with a child who has motion sickness, encourage her to breathe out of her mouth and not her nose. Also, move to the center of the boat (being on the bow and stern can aggravate motion sickness). Sometimes an ice pack or a cool washcloth on the back of the neck can help ease symptoms.

Zoos

You belong in the zoo! Zoos are a great place for your toddler and for you. They are educational, it's exciting to see all the animals and learn about them, and it's good exercise to walk through the park. The usual things that can set off a meltdown are if your toddler is tired, teething, hungry, or hot or cold. Zoos are known to be kid friendly, so you can let your toddler explore and play a bit more than you could in the local Target. As always, be prepared to take breaks, get snacks, and have some quiet time if needed. Try and catch an animal show while you're there, but if your toddler has a difficult time sitting through activities, find seating at the end of the row and close to an exit in case you need to make a hasty mid-show getaway.

Play

Now that your toddler is growing up, he is beginning to play differently with other children his age. He will slowly begin to want to share his things, and even when he doesn't, this is a good teaching moment for you as the parent or caregiver to demonstrate good ways to share and trade toys together. Children will start out playing beside another peer and then slowly begin to interact with the other child in their play, which is known as *cooperative interaction.* He begins to realize that other people (children and adults) can have impact on his idea of playing with a particular toy.

Play can be many things: creative, exploratory, and sometimes even competitive. Your child will most likely play anytime, anywhere. Let him. Play with him in the car, at the store, and while waiting for your food in the restaurant. Why? Because play is a wonderful way to communicate with your child. Not all of life is a game, but learning how to deal with life takes imagination to create solutions, develop the ability to make choices and the skill to take turns, and communicate. Therefore, play is extremely useful in most life situations. Engaging your toddler in play encourages him to be a thinker. So much of life for a toddler is about limitations and rules, but during play, he's encouraged to expand his mind and assert his individualism.[9]

There are many ways to foster communication during play with your child. For example, you can make up a story together. You can start, and then ask your child to chime in, such as, "Teddy bear wants to go play, he's going to go out all by himself. Should teddy bear run across the street or should he use the crosswalk?" Your child may be silly and say, "Run across the street!" And you can say, "Oh no, is he going to be hit by a car?" And you can talk about taking the bear to the hospital. Have fun and find the lessons in play while being silly.

Most importantly, see if your child is processing what he is taking in. Does your child understand you? Is he able to speak three-word sentences? Does he look at you when you talk? Is he distracted by clocks ticking or by people's cell phones ringing in the restaurant? Use play to make sure that your child's sensory systems are developing correctly. Does your child fall down a lot while playing? Does he misjudge the distance between his feet and the steps? Does he put toys on the coffee table to look at and focus his vision?

Dads

Make sure that your child's father is making time for play, whether he lives with the child or lives elsewhere. While dads are famous for their roughhousing, wrestling skills, and throwing kids around in the pool, they're also good male role models. It can be hard to find time for Daddy to play with a toddler after a long day of work, but maybe they can walk the dog together in the evenings. Dad could be in charge of the nightly bath, making bubbles and sinking ships with your little one. Dad and your toddler could have a standing breakfast date on Saturday mornings at the pancake house. What's better than Dad time and smiley-face pancakes? The point is to keep open lines of communication so that as your child grows, she will feel comfortable coming to Dad for advice and support instead of just thinking of him as the grouch on the couch she spends a week of vacation time with in the summer.

If your child's father is not in the picture or you have adopted your child as a single parent, try and have an uncle be a part or your child's life, or a friend or coworker that you are close to. Grandpas can be loads of fun, too. You can always be a part of the playdate too, if you're not comfortable leaving your little one with a male surrogate. Meet at the park, and while your child plays, you can catch up on the calls you've been wanting to make or read a book. You'll be there, but not exactly participating or hovering.

Rules

Play doesn't have to involve following the rules! My son really liked to make up his own games and rules, which some kids went along with and others did not. Often parents will play the part of referee amongst children playing; however, it's important to explain that no child is necessarily *wrong,* they're just wanting to play different games. It isn't until a child is older that she can really understand and follow all the rules. If you want to play Monopoly by the book, perhaps you should wait until the kids are in bed. If you expect a toddler to be able to sit there as you build hotels on Park Place, good luck with that.

Your toddler might also be rigid when it comes to the games that she's making up—who can play and how it is done. While this doesn't seem like a serious issue now, you may want to ease her into adjusting to the correct rules sometimes so that she's able to transition and be flexible when she's expected to play with peers as she gets older. An easy way to do that is to say, "Wow, Tiffany, those are some cool rules you've come up with. This is what the directions say, and the way that you would play with your friends." She doesn't have to play that way right now, but it's good for her to at least know there are rules to follow down the road.

Rules that pertain to safety are obviously completely different. When it says, "No diving in the shallow end of the pool," then there is NO diving in the shallow end. If your child is having difficulties following the rules when safety is an issue, either remove her from the situation or explain that she may not get into the pool unless she follows the rules. Give her a choice that you can follow through with. Follow the rules or go home.

It's completely possible to be safe *and* have fun!

Parents' Role in Play

You do not have to play with your child every second of every day, and you also don't want to play with your child only once a week. Moderation is key and allowing her to learn to play by herself is important, too. Know that your child is going to be asserting her authority at this age. She's going to say no, can be bossy, and may have monumental meltdowns. Toddlers needs lots of cuddle time to recuperate from play and tantrums. Make sure you supply ample hugs and squeezes to support her through this learning process.

Toddlers are not hung up on gender roles, as adults are. They may play superhero and princess and everything in between with each other, and they don't care if their playdates are with boys or girls. Many boys like the feel of princess dresses and want to try on Cinderella's sparkling shoes. So what? They're pretty. This does not mean your son is going to want to wear pink shoes to school. Remember, they're explorers at this age. Don't be hard on your toddler when it comes to "being a man." Whether you want your daughter to be the next Hilary Clinton or Sarah Palin or somewhere in between, pushing her to be in beauty pageants when she wants to play in the mud is not going to get either of you anywhere. Princess movies will not make your child forego college in the hopes of finding Prince Charming. Embrace what your child is interested in and what she gravitates toward.

Don't be the pushy parent who always expects her child to be the best. Whether he wins or loses is okay, as long as he tries his best. Find your child's strengths and help him to excel in a particular area if that is important to you, but don't resort to name-calling or ridicule, such as "Don't be a scaredy-cat" or "When I was your age, I could score 10 goals a game!" Sarcasm and what you might consider light-hearted joking can be belittling for a child. Many children already feel powerless and judged throughout the day, whether it be at daycare or preschool or with their older siblings or cousins. Empower your child so that he may excel in the future.

Play can be emotional for both you and your toddler. Examine and learn to control emotions through play. For example, make a tent and be scared with your child as you pretend you're camping in the desert and hear coyotes howling. Be sad with your child while pretending that you didn't get to go to a birthday party. You can be "pretend angry" with your child, too, but with all these pretend games, make sure your child knows that you are playing and not really mad at him. These exercises help your child to learn how to calm himself down while he's feeling these emotions and also to learn how to react in these situations. Show him how to switch emotional gears. Be sad, then happy, then frightened, then sad in a matter of moments. Always finish with laughter and find a peaceful center. This will help your child relieve stress and pent-up emotions and learn that it is okay to feel negative emotions and that there are ways to control them.

Funsucker

If there is one thing you not want to be known as to your friends, it is a "funsucker"—someone who takes the fun out of any and every situation. Life isn't perfect, so don't try to force it to be or try to make your kids perfect. Let them make mistakes, even in play. Don't turn every moment into a photo opportunity. Snap your shots at a designated area or time and then get on with your day, or take a million photos during the day and only keep the good ones. Take silly shots on your digital camera, too, and show your toddler—she'll think outrageous photos of herself are hilarious!

Roughhousing

Wrestling and roughhousing are a normal part of development. Both boys and girls will enjoy a good rough and tumble with Daddy, usually right before bedtime—exactly when you DON'T want them to get riled up. According to Dr Lawrence J. Cohen, author of *Playful Parenting,* wrestling helps children test their physical strength, control their anger, and learn physical boundaries.[10] Many children will experiment with wrestling, hitting, and pulling before trying out their skills on their peers in rough play.

Keep your rough play sessions short and stop immediately if anyone gets hurt. Let your toddler know it's not okay to hurt Daddy, either—he can assert himself but needs to learn how to control himself. Make sure he understands that there is no biting, hair-pulling, or foul play in wrestle time. It's more of a proprioceptive exercise, if you will, by providing just the right level of resistance for both you and the child.

Pay close attention to whether your child is getting too aggressive or out of control. If he is, stop immediately. Tickling is not allowed in roughhousing play, as it evokes the feeling of being out of control, which is the opposite lesson you are teaching during roughhouse play.

It's a good idea to cuddle afterward, to keep your parent-child connection strong and to let your child know that you are both okay. Snuggle together on the couch while watching a DVD or reading a book together. Always end on a positive note.

Pretend Play

Children will begin pretend play between 2 and 3 years, and items will begin to symbolize something. A cardboard box might be a castle, or a teddy bear in a blanket may be your toddler's baby. Her imagination may be taking off, or she might need some help from you to unlock her creativity. Have fun with this. What you are witnessing is your child processing all the millions of pieces of information that she takes in every day and making sense of it all.

Fisher-Price's Little People or any people toys, action figures, dolls, and stuffed animals are great for children to explore their surroundings and learn about the world we live in. Get down on the floor and create situations with your child, or, if she wants to set it up herself, observe if she's talking out loud to herself. Are her Little People having conversations? Is she figuring out how to solve a problem like a flat tire or deciding to have peanut butter and jelly sandwiches for lunch? Is one stuffed baby elephant getting in trouble by G.I. Joe? You can learn a lot about what your child is thinking and how she's feeling if you pay attention. Is she feeling left out in preschool? Did she have a bad day with the nanny and get scolded? Did her older brother pull her ponytail? Is she scared of the dark and going to bed? She may reenact these situations as she organizes them in her mental filing system.

Playing House

Playing "Mommy" and "Daddy" is super fun for toddlers! Oh how exciting it would be to be the boss of everyone and to take care of a baby. Of course, her baby isn't crying or filling a diaper. Is your daughter acting really bossy and mean to her baby? She might be experimenting with her authority, but also take a step back and see if she's mimicking you. Is it time for a mommy tune-up? Or is she roaring like Daddy that the baby is a pain in the neck? Yes, she does hear everything, even if she acts like she's ignoring us.

It is okay for the mommy/daddy roles to be reversed, as she is not completely clear about gender differences at this age. If you're breastfeeding a baby while your son is a toddler, he may breastfeed his baby doll. Do not read into this as weird or something to worry about—your son simply doesn't know that men do not process milk, and he's curious about how mommy feeds the baby. This will pass.

If you are a working parent, your child might pretend he's going to work himself and say good-bye to you as he carries his makeshift briefcase.

Pretend Kitchen

There are many play kitchens on the market, and it's no wonder—toddlers love them! It's so much fun to control an area that they're usually shooshed out of. They get to master the stove that is usually too hot for them and are able to use "knives" to cut plastic fruit. These kitchens are usually a good investment, because once they tire of playing kitchen, it turns into a drive-through restaurant! Endless possibilities of play come out in kitchen games, which work many different sensory systems. Use her play kitchen to introduce new foods to your toddler. Ask her about items she'd like to purchase from the grocery store and make a list together. (Remember, real food goes bad quickly! Don't leave eggs in the pretend refrigerator!)

School

If your child is in daycare, she most likely plays "school" with peers already. At home, she might be anticipating school and the excitement of the classroom. Playing school is a common theme amongst toddlers, where they get to be the teacher and control the situation. Your child is preparing herself for her next occupation—being a student—which will last through high school. You are able to answer some of her questions about school through play and ease any fears. Talk about how fun recess will be with her friends and all the fun art projects she will be making. Practice taking pretend tests and being still during story time. Most kids need to learn to quiet themselves at the appropriate lesson times. This can be a difficult task to master. Make it a competition. Can Mommy be still longer than Billy? Don't forget to raise your hand to ask a question!

Doctor Visit

Most children will play "going to visit the doctor and dentist." This may be a way to learn how to get through a scary appointment that is coming up or perhaps processing their last visit, which may or may not have been painful. At this age, they still don't know how to express that their teeth may be sensitive or that the lights reflecting off the dentist's glasses hurt their eyes. Pay attention to what your toddler says during these reenactments. Is she worried about receiving a shot? Or maybe the doctor's hands are cold, and it scares her. She might just need to work through her overall anxiety of not knowing what the dentist is going to do with those frightening tools on the tray.

Developmentally Appropriate Toys:
2 to 3 Years

Any sort of craft/coloring project is great. Markers and crayons are always fun, and you can begin helping him cut with safety scissors around $2^{1}/_{2}$ or 3 years of age, depending on his level of interest. Make sure you supervise him at all times when using safety scissors, as many children have given themselves a haircut!

- *An easel with finger paints.* Some children prefer easels because the slant positioning can be more comfortable and provides support for weak wrists and hands. It may be easier for them to see their artwork, since it is closer to their faces than a paper lying flat on the table.

- *Stringing beads and pasta.* Macaroni necklaces strung with yarn will be magnificent jewelry that your child can make you for Mother's Day. Work on her fine-motor skills by stringing large beads and pasta of various shapes, as well as lacing cards.

- *Puzzles that are age appropriate.* Puzzles get more complex as your child gets older. Make sure you're matching her skill level with her ability. You want it to be challenging, but not so much that she gets frustrated and gives up.

- *Mini-trampoline* (always use with supervision).

- *Jumping is a big skill for kids to learn and master.* Remember, both feet are off the ground! If your child finds this task difficult, help him hold onto the rail while he jumps. He may just bend his knees and bounce at first. If he's fearful or unable to lift both feet off the ground at once, he may have a gravitational insecurity. Has he had an ear infection recently? Maybe his inner-ear fluid is blocked and is causing him to feel unstable.

When he does jump, the trampoline provides proprioceptive feedback from the feet, up through the body, and all the way to the head. Jumping will help him regulate himself, so keep encouraging him to practice. Pretend to be frogs or Tigger on the ground, if the trampoline is too much for him!

- *Swings.* Both indoor and outdoor swings are good for kids because they get the inner-ear fluids moving, which stimulates the vestibular system. Be sure to swing linearly, meaning front to back. If you spin the swing, be sure to wind one way and then unwind it to help your child regulate. Don't force your child to spin if she doesn't like it, and stop the spinning if she gets dizzy. Watch for color changes in your child's face if she is getting too much vestibular input on the swing or other equipment.

- *Slides.* Climbing up and then sliding down—oh life is good when you're two. Again, this works the vestibular system by moving the fluids in the inner ear, as well working on gross-motor skills and bilateral coordination.

- *Tunnels.* Kids enjoy crawling through tunnels. You can find these at some parks, purchase them, or make your own out of a Lycra type of material. The Lycra tunnel will give your child immense proprioceptive feedback, and he will be using reasoning skills to figure out how to find the opening and crawl out of the tunnel.

- *Pretend tool set.* Many kids like to fix things. These tool kits make them feel empowered to take matters into their own little hands. Besides being fun, they're confidence and self-esteem builders. Turning a screw and hammering nails also help perfect fine-motor skills and hand-eye coordination.

- *A play piano and other musical instruments.* The banging on musical instruments might make you a little bonkers, but your child will be delighted to control the keyboard and her fingers, loudly sending musical notes into the stratosphere.

- *Building blocks and Legos.* There is something magical about building. It unlocks the imagination, logic and reasoning skills, sequencing, problem-solving, cause and effect, and trial and error. Simple blocks are all a child needs, but the many worlds that can be built with Legos are engaging and complex. Pay attention to how your child reacts to building. Is he obsessive about it? Does he fall apart if the building isn't perfect and destroy it? Does he have a tantrum if anyone touches the blocks that he's lined up? Help him to learn that the more he practices, the better he will be able to build. Perhaps you can find a spot for him to build where he can keep his structures up for a few days, and then give him a warning before it's time to put them away so he can transition.

- *Basketball, soccer ball, and football.* Break out the sports. While your child might not grasp all the rules of these games, he's most likely interested if you watch sports on TV or attend live sporting events. Both girls and boys benefit from exercise outdoors, the interaction with peers and adults, and utilizing their gross-motor muscle groups. If your child does not like sports, dig deeper to find out why. Is it that she doesn't like people running toward her? Is he scared of the physical impact when tackled? Is it impossible for her to throw the ball forward? Does he always miss the ball when he tries to kick it? This could be a sensory issue or a combination of sensory issues.

- *Play-Doh and Moon Sand* (supervise during the use of both, please!). We have posted instructions on how to make your own "gak," a fun coagulated goo, on our Web site *(www.TRPwellness.com)*. These doughlike items are wonderful for strengthening hands and wrists, all the way up the arm and into the shoulder, which helps build strength for writing. If your child doesn't like the feel of these items, ease her into playing with them by letting her wear gloves or plastic bags on her hands.

- *Obstacle course.* Playing "Follow the Leader" during an obstacle course will develop your child's ability to organize his behavior. That translates to being able to transition from one activity to the next, follow directions, remember patterns, and calm himself down. You can do this in your home or outside. Have your child follow you as you crab-walk from the kitchen to the living room, jump three times in place, then crawl through a tunnel while pushing a ball. If you're at the park, have him climb the ladder, slide down the slide, and then bear-walk through the sand to the merry-go-round. You get the idea. Repeat the sequence a few times. Your child may want to be the leader or take turns being the leader. Make it interesting, and remember—it's always okay to be silly. Other kids from the park may want to join in the fun.

Developmental Milestones, 2 to 3 Years

24-25 MONTHS

Gross- and Fine-Motor Development

- Runs well, without falling as much
- Walks up stairs alone
- Kicks a large ball
- Stands on tiptoes
- Pulls toy while walking
- Climbs onto and off of furniture without help
- Scribbles spontaneously
- Unwraps some food items
- Imitates a circle
- Might use one hand more frequently than the other (but hand preference can take up until the age of 5 or 6 to be decided, so don't worry if your child switches back and forth)

Visual Development

- Throws a large ball
- Kicks a ball forward

Speech and Language Development

- Understands the difference between "in/on," "go/stop," "big/little," and "up/down"
- Follows a two-step direction ("Go get your shoes and bring them to me.")
- Has a word for almost everything
- Uses two- to three-word sentences

Social and Cognitive Development

- Finds objects even when hidden
- Begins to sort items by shape and color
- Imitates the behavior of others

- Defends possessions
- Throws more frustration-based tantrums between 24 and 30 months
- Takes pride in getting self dressed
- Uses the word "mine" for property
- Puts shoes on with assistance
- Holds a small cup with one hand
- Unbuttons large buttons
- Helps put things away
- Pulls pants down with assistance

26-30 MONTHS

Gross- and Fine-Motor Development
- Walks down stairs alone
- Enjoys jumping
- Holds crayon in fingers rather than fist
- Removes pants and pulls down undergarments
- Builds a block tower of at least eight to ten blocks

Visual Development
- Catches a large ball thrown gently to him
- Makes small cuts with child-safe scissors and some help

Speech and Language Development
- Labels objects, animals, and colors
- Points to an object in a picture when it's named

Social and Cognitive Development
- Fatigues easily
- Holds a parent's hand outdoors
- Tends to be physically aggressive
- Becomes aware of differences in sex
- Begins make-believe play
- Displays shyness toward strangers
- Washes hands

- Holds spoon in fingers, is able so eat with a spoon and fork
- Undresses with a little assistance
- Rejects many food items (sometimes in phases)

30-36 MONTHS

Gross- and Fine-Motor Development
- Rides a tricycle
- Climbs a lot
- Balances on one foot briefly
- Throws a ball overhand
- Jumps with both feet
- Copies a circle well
- Feeds self independently
- Uses scissors but doesn't necessarily cut on the line
- Unlaces shoes
- Snaps front snaps
- Holds a crayon well

Visual Development
- Pours liquid from a container into a cup

Speech and Language Development
- Asks short questions
- Repeats simple rhymes
- Talks about feelings
- Knows his first and last name
- Knows whether he/she is a boy or a girl
- Tries to make others laugh

Social and Cognitive Development
- Begins to obey and respect simple rules
- Resists change
- Has difficulty with transitions
- Tends to be demanding, thinks the world centers around him

- Separates easily from his mother in a familiar setting
- Helps with bathing himself
- Hangs clothing on a hook
- Can put on a shirt that buttons in front (although he cannot manage the buttons yet)
- Verbalizes a need to use the toilet
- May awaken in the night from dreams
- May begin to eliminate naps

Evaluating Your Child's Senses

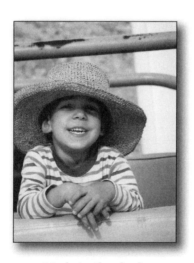

Made in the shade.
QUINTIN, 2 YEARS OLD

Is Your Child Hyper- or Hyposensitive?

HYPERSENSITIVE MEANS THAT YOUR BABY OR TODDLER IS OVERRESPONSIVE to certain sensory input. *Hyposensitive* means that your baby or toddler is underresponsive to sensory input. According to Dr Lucy Jane Miller, "We hypothesize that a child with overresponsiveness has a low threshold for sensation. He feels things too soon, too much. He may be sensitive to loud sounds, even when you may not think they are that loud. We also hypothesize that a child with underresponsiveness has a high threshold for sensation. He feels things too late, too little. He doesn't hear someone calling his name, and he doesn't feel the 'owie.'"

Signs of Hypersensitivity

- Covering his ears to avoid certain sounds
- Overreacting to various temperatures (either feeling really cold or really hot when you may think the temperature is average)
- Screaming or picking up his feet when you place him in the grass barefoot
- Not wanting any messy food on his face or not wanting to touch anything sticky or gooey
- Spitting out textured food because he can't tolerate the way it feels
- Getting scared, crying, or clinging to you when you toss your child in the air
- Looking terrified, crying, or clinging to you when you place your child in a swing
- Is bothered by movement—he doesn't like to jump, skip, or hop
- Pulls away to avoid being touched

Signs of Hyposensitivity

- Craves a lot of deep pressure, crashes into the couch and furniture, gives hard high fives, gives really strong, hard hugs
- Moves all the time, can't remain still, fidgets and wiggles and darts around the room
- Loves to spin
- Falls down and doesn't cry when it looks like he should be hurt
- Has a high tolerance for pain

- Loves hot and spicy foods because he may not really taste what's in his mouth
- Is always placing his hands in his mouth or stuffing food in his mouth
- Grinds his teeth, seeks out deep pressure in the mouth
- Jumps a lot
- Doesn't hear his name when called
- Is lethargic or habitually doesn't want move off the couch (has no inner drive to move)
- May not be able to tell whether bath water is too hot or too cold
- Drools a lot or loses food when eating after about 24 months

Here are some more examples to consider. Your child may be *hypersensitive or overresponsive* if she does not want to wear clothes or if she only wants to wear one particular outfit that is soft and loose. Maybe she can't tolerate walking barefoot and insists on wearing shoes or has you put a blanket down for her to walk on. There also may be times when she never wants to wear socks or shoes because they feel too constricting on her feet. If she can't even touch spaghetti noodles or other foods with her fingers, then she's hypersensitive. She may also be sensitive to movement— for instance, riding in an elevator could send her into a crying frenzy. These children are in "fight, flight, or freeze" mode most of the time.

Hyposensitive means that your baby or toddler is underresponsive to input. He may not notice if the bath water is too hot or too cold. He may fall down and not cry or come tell you that he hurt himself. A child that is underresponsive is more sedentary than a typically developing child and may not like to move as much because his body takes a lot of input to register what he is feeling. These children are not always aware of their surroundings.

What if your child is both hyper- *and* hyposensitive? What if some days she's fine, and other days she's lethargic half the time and hyper the other half? Then what?! Fortunately, you're not alone. After reading Carol Kranowitz's book, *The Out-of-Sync Child,* I learned that it is possible for a child to be both hyper- and hyposensitive.[11] I also learned how to better detect a sensory-processing issue. Whether your child is hyper- or hyposensitive, there are things you can work on to help your child's sensory needs.

In the latest research by Dr Lucy Jane Miller, she poses that in addition to overresponsive and underresponsive children, you also have those children who are always moving, or "on the go." She calls this category "sensory seekers and cravers." These children constantly respond to every new sensory stimulus that they come into contact with. For example, a child that likes to spin constantly is seeking out this input, but from an occupational therapist's viewpoint, we don't want to give him more of this spinning movement because it could make him more disorganized or "hyperactive."

It is a normal desire to seek out a hot shower on a cold day or to want chewing gum to satisfy an oral craving. These are ways of seeking out sensation and satisfying our need for it. The problem is when a child is seeking more input that what is typical. Here are some signs that your child might be a sensory seeker or craver.

Signs of Sensory Seekers and Cravers

- Likes deep pressure, crashes into the couch and furniture, gives hard high fives, gives really strong, hard hugs
- Moves all the time, can't remain still, fidgets and wiggles and darts around the room
- Loves to spin
- Grinds his teeth, seeks out deep pressure in the mouth
- Puts nonfood objects in his mouth past an appropriate age of around 12 months
- Jumps a lot
- May also love hot and spicy foods with a lot of flavor
- Is in fast-blast mode, running into people and objects and not paying attention to his surroundings because he cannot slow his body down.

If you notice that your child is having a difficult time functioning, and you think it is possibly due to sensory issues, you may want to seek out an occupational therapist to help you evaluate what your child's specific sensory needs are and learn about how to help her regulate herself.

If your child seeks out a lot of crashing, gives hard high fives, spins a lot without getting dizzy, is always running, and runs into walls and coffee tables as though she doesn't see them, she may have some vestibular and proprioceptive difficulties. An occupational therapist trained in sensory integration can help evaluate your child and come up with a sensory diet for you to do daily with your child to give her deep-pressure input, heavy-work activities, vestibular activities, and more to help her regulate her system. This may include having your child carry your laundry basket full of clothes into the bedrooms where you're putting the clothes away (heavy work). Or, an occupational therapist may have your child jump on a mini-trampoline to get proprioceptive and vestibular input, which will help regulate her internal systems throughout the day.

Tactile Example: Therapeutic Brushing Techniques

When a child is tactile defensive and doesn't want to walk barefoot on various textures, has a hard time tolerating clothing textures, won't touch anything gooey or sticky, and hates having his hair washed and his teeth brushed, you may want to consider implementing a skin-brushing program, called the Wilbarger Deep Pressure and Proprioceptive Technique and Oral Tactile Technique. The technique was developed by Patricia Wilbarger, MEd, OTR, FAOTA, who is an occupational therapist and clinical psychologist also known for coining the phrase "sensory diet."[12] This program can only be taught to you by a trained professional. While the focus appears to be on the surgical brush on the skin, it's actually more about the deep pressure from the brush and the gentle compressions after the brushing, which provide substantial proprioceptive input. You will learn that the face and stomach are NEVER brushed. Occupational therapists are primarily the ones who have been trained in this program. The skin is your largest organ, and when you brush the skin, you are bringing increased awareness to your body. Children may become more tolerant of various textures, as well as demonstrate increased balance, coordination, and body awareness. This protocol must be strictly monitored by an occupational therapist.

MOM EXAMPLE: The Wilbarger brushing protocol worked well with my son, as he couldn't tolerate it when I applied sunscreen to his skin. After months of following the protocol, I was able to apply sunscreen without causing a wrestling match and a tantrum.

Will He/She Grow Out of It? What If I Ignore It?

Most of the time, we as humans learn how to deal with sensory sensitivities, or we make adaptations, or we avoid situations that we know will make us uncomfortable. For instance, I am overly sensitive to auditory sounds. I do not *like* the sound of the dishwasher or the washing machine running, but can I tolerate it if I have to? Yes! Would I rather run those machines when I am not home or far enough away in another room so I cannot hear them? Absolutely.

When a child is having a sensory issue, I ALWAYS address it. Sometimes it is hard to tell whether it's a sensory issue or a behavioral one. Is your child throwing tantrums at daycare because he wants to be at home, or is it a sensory issue? Does your child get overwhelmed with too many children around him? Is your child able to block out some of the noise of the other children, or is he having auditory issues? Is the daycare provider's perfume potent and offensive to your child's sensory system? Sometimes it takes a trained eye to be able to tell the difference, and you should react differently according to the situation. If your child seems to be throwing tantrums more than other toddlers, and you are not able to identify to reason behind them, talk to your pediatrician about an occupational therapy evaluation to see if there are underlying sensory needs that need to be addressed. Occupational therapists can also help give you tips to get the behaviors under control. Now as we know, most toddlers are going to fuss and cry when they don't get their way, but they should not be doing this every day, and they should not be throwing themselves down on the floor every time you tell them they cannot have a piece of candy.

As a parent, you need to remember that everyone processes sensory information differently, and when we have sensitivities to certain sensory input, we all react differently.

Occupational Therapy and Sensory Integration

So, what exactly is an occupational therapist? Well, we work with people of all ages, from birth until the time of death. You may see an occupational therapist in a hospital setting, a school, a home, a skilled nursing facility, or an outpatient clinic. When working with children, we see all sorts of conditions, including autism spectrum disorders, Down syndrome, cerebral palsy, developmental delays, SPD, brain injury, spina bifida, and more. We focus on improving the quality of life and improving the functional skills required for everyday living. If an adult has recently had a stroke or lost a limb, occupational therapists reteach them how to cook, get dressed, possibly go back to work, drive, and do many other things. When people have gone through a traumatic life change, they need to learn a whole new way of living and adapting, and an occupational therapist is taught how to do that. We're usually quite creative and are knowledgeable about adaptations and modifications.

I (Britt) am a pediatric occupational therapist, and I currently work in a hospital. My daily patients include children with Down syndrome, cerebral palsy, autism spectrum disorders, attention-deficit/hyperactivity disorder, and SPDs; paraplegics; drug-affected children; and many,

many more. My goal is to motivate them to be independent with their daily-living skills, to use sensory integration to help them process their daily sensory input, and to teach parents adoptive strategies. I have also worked in a school setting, where we focus on helping the children to process their senses in the school environment and come up with adaptations to foster independence and set up a successful school career. In a private clinic or home setting, I work primarily on introducing sensory diets into the home and community so that a child is able to regulate himself and process all necessary sensory information. I also work on gross-, fine-, and visual-motor skills and help children with skills such as writing, cutting, dressing, and even riding a bike.

If you have concerns about your child's sensory-processing abilities, here are some examples of what an occupational therapist may do to provide sensory-integration therapy.

Example Client A

A 3-year-old child has gross-motor delays, fine-motor delays, and tactile defensiveness. An occupational therapist may *(a)* focus on strengthening her core muscles, *(b)* work on catching and throwing a ball, *(c)* assist the child with sitting and working on drawing simple shapes, *(d)* encourage playing with Play-Doh and shaving cream, *(e)* set up a home program for the family to implement at home, and more.

Example Client B

A 4-year-old child has autism and severe sensory issues, which lead to having tantrums multiple times a day. He is unable to transition from a preferred to a nonpreferred task and is unable to tolerate any sort of movement. The occupational therapist may focus on slowly introducing a swing and picking him up and putting him down to get vestibular input. She may also give him a weighted vest to wear to help calm him down and increase his tolerance to transition. She would encourage transitioning between two preferred activities and work up to transitioning from a preferred activity to a nonpreferred activity. Reinforcement would be provided with positive verbal reinforcement and maybe toys or stickers. She might work on dressing skills and writing skills with him, as well.

The list can go on, but this gives you a small insight into how occupational therapy could help your child if he is having any of the issues we have talked about in this book.

Sensory Processing Disorder

By now, you're either familiar with sensory integration or you're wondering what, exactly, we're talking about! *Sensory integration dysfunction* was coined by the late (and we think really great) developmental psychologist, Dr A. Jean Ayres. The term refers to the seven senses and their level of efficiently organizing information in the brain and throughout the nervous system. While there is still an incredible amount of research to be done on the subject, Jean Ayres pioneered the occupational treatments that help correct this disorder. Whether your baby has sensory dysfunction or just needs a little redirection or reprogramming, we're grateful for the doors that have opened as a result of learning about sensory integration, and we hope to continue carrying the torch to help ourselves and others. The common term used now is *sensory processing disorder,* or SPD.

You may wonder, "What does my child not liking tags in his shirt have to do with anything?" Or, "Why should it matter if he's hyposensitive and rough, he'll make a great football player!" These things matter because disorders of sensory processing transfer into all aspects of your child's life, including how he plays with others (or can't play with others), how he learns in school (or can't learn, because of processing dysfunctions), and how he grows up and becomes an active, fulfilled adult who participates in society and performs an occupation he excels at (or if he can't!). When a child is not able to process the sensory information he's receiving, it affects his emotional state of being and may cause anxiety, insecurities, and depression. If he's uncomfortable in a hectic environment, on the playground, and in the classroom, then this will affect his ability to make friends and have healthy relationships. When a child has physical processing issues that affect the way he walks, and if he's running into things, then he will most likely avoid being around other children and feel embarrassed when he's labeled as clumsy or awkward.

Dr Lucy Jane Miller, PhD, OTR, founder of the SPD Foundation and author of *Sensational Kids,* notes that at least one in 20 people in the general population is affected by SPD.[13] Occupational therapists may specialize in sensory integration and aid in reteaching the brain how to process the multisensory information that it takes to do everything in life. They help with desensitization, organizing of behavior, sequencing, calming the body, and many, many other things. The science behind SPD is still being actively researched and studied, but many have experienced remarkable results.

Occupational therapist Lindsey Biel, coauthor of *Raising a Sensory Smart Child: The Definitive Handbook for Helping Your Child with Sensory Processing Issues,* writes extensively about the importance of a sensory diet for a child with SPD.[14] She encourages providing active occupational therapy for the child, as well as parent input, throughout the day to empower the child and encourage independence. She provides many practical solutions and activities to incorporate into daily life in her book and DVD (Sensory Processing Masterclass), on her Web site (*sensorysmarts.com*), in featured articles, and at conferences and clinics nationwide.

As an occupational therapist and mom team, we encourage you to work with your occupational therapist on what is best for your child. Also, educate yourself about SPD as much as possible by reading the remarkable books that are out there, so that you may carry on a comprehensive conversation with your child's early-intervention team and come up with ideas to help your child at home, in school, and in your local environment.

Maybe after reading this, you'll realize that you may have more sensory-processing dysfunction than you were aware of! Do you avoid crowded movie theaters, the mall, and grocery stores during peak hours? Or do you seek out activities where you receive a rush, like riding roller coasters or jumping from an airplane? Do clothes and shoes feel uncomfortable and distract you throughout the day? Are you unable to concentrate at work if your office neighbor is playing music on his computer? Winnie Dunn has written a book called *Living Sensationally* for those of you who would like to further understand the type of sensory processor you are (or maybe what type your spouse is). It's amazing how much easier it is to understand people in general when you see how there are subgroups and types of processors. There is also a book by Dr Sharon Heller, *Too Loud, Too Bright, Too Fast, Too Tight,* for those of you who have had a traumatic accident or have gotten increasingly sensory sensitive as you have aged. It can be painful and scary to grow increasingly sensitive to lights, sounds, tastes, and touch, but it can also be pretty common. If a hug or physical contact is painful or uncomfortable, seek out an occupational therapist in your area to help relieve your symptoms.

The bottom line is this: There is help out there for you and your child! Go get it—you will be glad you did. Attend a sensory conference in your town or in a town you'd like to visit. Read books, search the Web, become an expert on yourself and your child. Join a support group and chat with others about what has worked for them and what hasn't. The sensory community is growing, and there are people out there who want to help you live your most comfortable, successful, and happy life.

Does My Child Have SPD, Autism, or ADHD?

Signs of SPD

My child:

- Is sensitive in one or more of the following areas, to the point of interfering with day-to-day functional skills: tactile, oral, vestibular (balance), proprioceptive (body awareness), auditory, visual, olfactory
- Is fearful of unexpected touch
- Is distressed during diaper changes
- Avoids certain textures

- Is excessively ticklish
- Refuses to have her teeth brushed, her nails cut, or her hair washed
- Is not aware of being touched
- Runs into things as if they are not there
- Craves a lot of deep pressure, gives hard high fives
- Prefers spicy, salty, or sweet foods
- Engages in self-abuse: hitting, biting, and/or pinching
- Avoids playground equipment (swings, slides, etc)
- Is afraid of heights, experiences fear when her feet leave the ground
- Cries when you lay her down in her crib and seems fearful that she is falling
- Has poor balance or is clumsy
- Is in constant motion, can't sit still
- Is impulsive (a thrill seeker)
- Rocks body or head while sitting
- Has limp, "floppy" body
- Gets tired easily
- Has difficulty getting dressed (in older children, has difficulty with buttons and zippers)
- Is unable to multitask
- Cannot transition from one activity to the next
- Has poor gross-motor skills (such as doing jumping jacks, riding a bike, going down the stairs one foot at a time)
- Grinds her teeth
- Is always putting things in her mouth
- Seems distressed by loud sounds (a fire alarm, a vacuum cleaner)
- Appears to make noise just to hear the noise she makes
- Covers her ears to avoid certain sounds

- Has difficulty transitioning from sleep to wakefulness and from wakefulness to sleep
- Gags on textured foods
- Is unable to try new textures of foods
- Licks or chews inedible objects past the appropriate oral-motor stage as an infant
- Avoids eye contact
- Plays in a dark room
- Is sensitive to bright lights
- Complains of seeing double
- Is unable to copy words from a chalkboard
- Has few social skills
- Prefers to play by herself
- Gets frustrated easily
- Is unable to imitate during play (after 10 months)

We talked to occupational therapist Emily Sylvester, who is certified in administering and interpreting the Sensory Integration Praxis Test, or SIPT. Emily currently lives in the Los Angeles area and works with children in an outpatient clinic setting and in a school setting. Emily has developed a strong focus on sensory integration through her occupational therapy work, which has led her to help children with various special needs, such as autism, attention-deficit/hyperactivity disorder, and cerebral palsy.

- *Do you work with typically developing children or only children with special needs?*

  I work with children of both populations, although I work with children with special needs more often.

- *How does an occupational therapist who specializes in sensory integration differ from a regular occupational therapist?*

An occupational therapist who specializes in sensory integration has a greater understanding of the underlying neurological and sensory-motor components that affect how people function and cope with the three-dimensional, tangible world. Sensory integration is a part of everyone's life, and occupational therapists who have expertise in sensory integration are able to identify and discriminate each sensory system, evaluate how they are relating to each other, and discern which systems are being processed and integrated poorly. It's our job to evaluate the client, come up with the best course of action, and provide a sensory diet.

- *What age groups do you work with?*

  I work with children aged 2 to 12.

- *How do you determine what type of sensory diet a child will need?*

  I take into consideration what sensory systems are overresponsive and underresponsive and what the child's present level of function is in the setting that the sensory diet will be used in.

- *If my child has SPD and I pick only one thing to work on, what would be the most important thing?*

  You need to choose whatever is most important to the child, the parent, and the family—there's never any *one* thing that is a first priority. As a therapist, you need to work within the values and priorities of the family you are working with. For example, if the family really struggles with the morning routine because of issues related to praxis and sensory processing, I would work on sensory-diet strategies and visuals for helping the child and other family members maintain an appropriate arousal level and sense of independence to alleviate the stress in the mornings.

- *What would you like to tell parents of children with SPD?*

  You are not alone. Stay positive throughout the process of helping your child with his or her SPD. Things can change, but don't expect changes to happen overnight!

Does My Child Have Autism?

The world of autism is confusing and complicated for parents to comprehend. It covers such a massive umbrella of diagnoses within the one label of autism: pervasive developmental disorder not otherwise specified, Asperger syndrome, low-, mild-, and high-functioning autism—I've even heard the term "autistic-like." While the trend was and may still be securing a diagnosis of autism to be able to receive services for your child, state and local government systems, school systems, and private practices are now so flooded that the autism label is no longer a magic pass into regional centers (state-run centers that offer services and resources for children with disabilities), early-intervention programs, insurance carriers, and school districts. Many children are now being described as "recovered," and some camps argue that those children didn't really have autism—perhaps they had sensory dysfunction and nutritional deficiencies. Other groups consider these children to be spoiled brats or difficult as a result of bad parenting, and some believe that those with severe autism are mentally retarded.

There have been major breakthroughs in autism awareness with movies like "Autism: The Musical," and Temple Grandin's life story, which aired on HBO; however, people are still unsure how to specifically define autism and, once diagnosed, how to go about treating and/or living with autism. As a new parent, you might be fearful that your child will catch autism, like the flu, or maybe you feel autism couldn't happen to you and your family. Following are some questions to ask yourself if you're exploring the possibility that autism is affecting your child.

Do you feel like something is "wrong?" Do you feel that your child is not like other children and doesn't fit in? Are you having a difficult time understanding what your baby wants and needs? Do you want to burn all the baby books that aren't giving you the guidance you need because your child doesn't fit into the category of baby they're talking about? Have you become overprotective of your child's behaviors? Do you make up excuses as to why your child is not developing at the same rate as other children?

Being that autism is on the rise and receiving media attention, more and more parents have the privilege of securing a diagnosis for their babies and toddlers and receiving early-intervention treatments. If you have any concerns, do not feel embarrassed or paranoid—have your child evaluated. If it turns out that your child does not have autism, and you feel silly for pushing for the tests, then congratulations! But if your child does have autism, early intervention can help, and the sooner you start getting the appropriate treatment for your child, the better.

Possible Signs of Autism

My child:

- Lines up toys
- Is unable to tolerate someone else playing with his toys or changing what he is doing
- Has difficulty transitioning from one activity to another
- Exhibits decreased eye contact
- Exhibits decreased language skills, has difficulty communicating (has few or no verbal skills)
- Is constantly repeating words or short groups of words or memorizing and repeating entire TV shows
- Cries and throws tantrums for no reason
- Shows little or no emotional connection with others
- Is unable to pretend-play
- Performs repeated body movements ("stimming," such as hand or arm flapping, rocking, hitting himself over and over again)
- Is a picky eater
- Has difficulty sleeping or transitioning from being awake to going to sleep
- Is fearful of people in general (at parks and family functions, in public, and at home)

- Is fearless (is completely unaware of any safety concerns or danger)
- Is overly fascinated and obsessed with one item or subject for an extended period

If your child exhibits several of these signs, you should talk to your pediatrician immediately and ask to make an appointment with a developmental pediatrician.

MOM TIP: There is a helpful checklist, M-CHAT, compiled by Diana Robins, Deborah Fein, and Marianne Barton, that is available online if you'd like to print a copy, fill it out, and share it with your pediatric physician as a starting point when discussing concerns you have about your child.

As a mother of a child with autism, other mothers who are going through similar experiences as me have been my sanctuary. They are where I find the most useful information, they have the strongest shoulders to cry on, and they offer the most unconditional friendship I've ever felt. When the professionals think you're crazy, overprotective, or downright ignorant, it is these fellow warrior moms who will take your call. Together, you will learn the vernacular to navigate through your child's therapies and treatments, and you will exchange crucial tips that will open doors and get your child through the regional centers, insurance plans, and school districts.

If your child receives a diagnosis of autism, I highly recommend joining an "autism mom group" immediately. It will be the best thing that you can do for yourself and your child. Andrea Lee is one of the mothers from the mom group that I joined upon my son's diagnosis. She is the mother of a beautiful autistic boy named Tyler. I cherish the invaluable information we have shared, the battles we have fought together on behalf of our children, and the camaraderie. I look forward to raising our sons together, because autism doesn't go away—it is here for both of our lifetimes.

This is what Andrea had to say about first learning that her son had autism.

Q&A with Andrea Lee

- *When did you first know your son had autism? What were the signs?*

You know what they say about hindsight being 20/20. For some parents of special-needs kids, the "moment" they knew is as clear as day, and they can single out that one incident, time, event, or feeling they had when they knew their child was not developing typically. It changes them and their lives forever. For me, looking back, I guess I always had a lingering and growing sense, a little signal inside my head or a gut feeling in my body that I ignored or pushed away. My son received an official diagnosis at 22 months and started receiving some treatment and services at close to 2 years of age, but as most moms will share, securing that diagnosis is often a long process. Getting someone to listen, getting your general pediatrician to refer you to a specialist, and waiting for the soonest appointment with the specialist all takes time and waiting. So in reality, I would say that I knew my son was not developing typically at around 1 year old—14 to 15 months. The signs were all there, but they were subtle and spread out and didn't happen all at once.

He was a healthy, happy baby who slept well, but around a year or so, there were signs: He made little or no eye contact and said no real words. In fact, he didn't really attempt simple words or sounds. There was no gesturing or pointing, and he did not imitate my sounds or gestures. Tyler was a lovely baby boy who seemed content, but I would say he was too content. He was with other babies and toddlers his age and seemed unfazed or disinterested in them and what they were doing. The toys or parts of toys were more fascinating than the kids around him. Left alone, autistic babies are almost too comfortable. Tyler did not care whether I was in the room or not, whether I walked away or came back, and there was no sense of clinginess or separation anxiety. As a first-time parent, I assumed he was a boy and self-reliant. I thought I was just fortunate to have a laid-back and content baby and toddler. In retrospect, however, these are signs that an autistic child is simply not engaged with people or capable of any form of verbal or nonverbal communication or interaction.

- *Was your pediatrician helpful or did you need to find new resources?*

My son's pediatrician was an older man, well educated, with a strong practice in Los Angeles. He came with excellent referrals and was kind, thoughtful, and cautious. For a typically developing baby and toddler, he would have been perfect. For an autistic kid, his approach can be disastrous. My pediatrician did not want to alarm me and quite frankly was not a developmental pediatrician who had great experience with or insight into autism. When I approached him at Tyler's 18-month checkup and said that I was concerned and wanted him to see a specialist, my pediatrician assured me that boys tend to take longer to verbalize words or be super social. He had me wait another 3 months, until Tyler was 21 months old, to even make a referral. He was trying to be calm and calm me down, but in the end, valuable time was wasted. After we got the referral and an official diagnosis at 22 months by a developmental pediatrician, we never really had a need to speak to him again, other than for regular health check-ups. General pediatricians become like ex-boyfriends. They are still around for health needs, such as the common cold and getting a flu shot and making sure your child is growing physically, but at that point, a parent with an autistic child must seek out a solid and competent developmental pediatrician who has experience with autism and can deal with all those challenges that become a bigger priority.

- *How do your son's sensory needs differ from those of typically developing children?*

  Parents have no idea how connected the sensory system is to autism in general, whether your child is mildly or greatly affected by sensory challenges. Tyler's autistic "symptoms" clearly decrease and increase according to the "regulation" of his body's sensory systems. If he is seeking deep pressure for his body, for example, he might be more hyper and jumpy and have difficulty remaining seated or keeping his arm from flapping. If the sun is bright and it agitates his eyes, then he may be more irritable and prone to having tantrums and meltdowns. When he was younger and he had poor muscle tone, especially around his mouth, it affected his eating and overall movement. Typically developing kids can have mild to severe sensory challenges too, but they are generally more isolated and can be treated more effectively. Occupational therapy and sensory integration can often be gradually phased out for those children, whereas an autistic child like Tyler will always have sensory issues that need to be addressed. He may improve over some months, and then there are times and seasons when he can regress and require more sensory-integration therapy.

- *What has been the biggest challenge in raising a son with autism?*

  The challenges are too many to count or measure, but I would say as a mother of an autistic son, the greatest challenge is the "not knowing"—the sense that there are no clear or definitive answers to any of the big questions all special-needs mothers and parents face. Is my son or daughter going to improve over time? Is the therapy I am using working? Will he or she be able to live independently one day? How will the world treat him? Will he be discriminated against? There are no answers to much of what parents must ask when they are seeking out medical and therapeutic interventions and making educational choices. A parent's overall anxiety and worry is magnified and increased many times over because autism is still a fairly new field. Much more money, time, and energy and many more resources are needed, not just for diagnosis and detection but for real, hands-on treatment that is effective. The financial burdens and expenses are crippling and can tear many families apart. It's emotionally challenging to care for a child whom you love desperately and want so much to help, at the same time knowing that many people, including professionals, school systems, therapists, and regular individuals, know very little in terms of how to deal with the individual needs of these children and adults. The unknown future and the realization that every day brings a new set of challenges and hurdles to overcome are sometimes daunting and unsettling.

- *What would you tell other parents of a child that recently received a diagnosis of autism?*

Tyler is now 7 years old, and my family and I have been dealing with his autism for more than 5 years. I tell a new mother or father to hang in there! I am not a religious person or one who ascribes to a certain set of beliefs, but I am spiritual and introspective and realized a long time ago that whoever decides your life or path doesn't give you what you simply can't bear. I would also recommend a very strong martini or a glass of red wine when the kids are in bed and you have a quiet moment! My husband gave me the best advice: Cry in the shower and never let your son or daughter see you hurting. Autistic kids are bright and super sensitive, and they pick up on your emotions and vibe. I would say that after the initial shock of a diagnosis, a decision must be made. Will you allow autism to bring you and your family down? Or will your rise above the label and the diagnosis and do the best you can with the resources you have? There are no guarantees in life, and the same can be said for these amazing children who WILL show you in unconventional ways and in the smallest gestures that they are capable and worthy and that they are to be celebrated and valued. So sip on that drink if you need it, soldier on, and do not leave any stone unturned. A parent can always be looking for better ways to help her autistic child. If something doesn't feel right, or you know that a therapist, a school, or a resource is not helping your child, then keep looking! 'No' is simply not an answer! It is exhausting and tiresome, but in the end, you'll feel great that you did all you could for your autistic child. It is a true disservice to yourself and to your child if you do not pursue every avenue that comes your way to help him improve his quality of life. And in the meanwhile, take the help and kindness of anyone who genuinely cares and wants to be in your child's life. You'll find it in the most unlikely places—a stranger's kind words, a store owner's patience, a grandparent's love. Wherever you might find it, it will make all the difference in the world.

Autism Resources

As a mother of a child with autism, I cannot express how important it is to educate yourself. There are extraordinary books and resources that will help you understand and seek services for your child. There is much to do, so get started immediately! Find the information and treatments that are best for you and your child, as every child with autism is unique. There is no "one size fits all" when it comes to the autism spectrum.

Future Horizons Publishing has a vast library of books, DVDs, and conferences on raising a child with autism. We highly recommend you start there *(www.fhautism.com)*. We have been buying their books and resources for years, and we are grateful for the knowledge they have provided and their dedication to serving the autism community.

Talk About Curing Autism, or TACA *(TACA.com), autismone.org,* and *autismspeaks.com* provide information, groups, and support at your fingertips.

Books we would recommend include *The First Year: Autism Spectrum Disorders: An Essential Guide for the Newly Diagnosed Child,* by Nancy D. Wiseman, and *Healing the New Childhood Epidemics Autism, ADHD, Asthma, and Allergies: The Groundbreaking Program for the 4-A Disorders,* by Kenneth Bock, MD, and Cameron Stauth.

Does My Child Have ADHD?

Attention-deficit/hyperactivity disorder, or ADHD, is another term that you might not have heard of before you had a baby, but you've likely been hearing all the buzz about it now. Like autism, ADHD has different levels and subtypes and a variety of treatments. Most are quick to medicate for this disorder, which can be positive for some kids and negative for others. Again, as a mother, I advise you to educate yourself and explore your options and various treatments for your child. Find out all the pros and cons of each medication, and talk to other parents with children who take these medications. What are the adverse health risks? What kind of reaction can you expect? What should you be looking for and monitoring?

I'm a big believer in searching for the underlying cause of any and all medical conditions. Can it be improved with diet and nutrition? Are there behavioral modifications and treatments you can try? Would sensory-integration therapy be effective? Or perhaps a combination of all of the above? Work with your developmental pediatrician and seek out a specialist who specifically treats children with ADHD.

Be an advocate for your child and make sure he's treated with respect in the school system. Even though he may be more difficult for the teacher to handle, he deserves a positive learning environment.

Signs of ADHD:

My child:

- Is hyperactive
- Is impulsive
- Has an inability to attend to a task, even for a few minutes
- Does not appear to hear you when you call his name or talk to him
- Has difficulty organizing tasks
- Often loses things (toys, school assignments, etc)
- Is easily distracted and has difficulty getting refocused on the task

Symptoms must be present for at least 6 months to warrant a diagnosis, and the symptoms must be observable in two or more settings. Some symptoms must be present before age 7, and they must be severe enough to cause significant difficulties with performing functional life skills.

Auditory Processing Disorder

Most babies and toddlers do not receive a diagnosis of auditory processing disorder until they're 2 ½ or 3 years old. This is mostly because a baby may pass the Apgar tests at birth and again pass hearing tests. How is it possible that a child with auditory processing disorder does not receive a diagnosis with these standard tests? Well, processing and hearing are not the same thing. Your child might hear a bell ring, but that does not mean that when you speak to him, his brain is processing and decoding this information in a comprehensible pattern. When a child is able to detect sound and yet he has auditory processing disorder, the mystery lies in where the problem originates. Is it in the various parts of the ear? Could it be the auditory nerve? Might the circuit be shorting in the central auditory pathways? Or could the malfunction be taking place when the information reaches the brain?

If your child has had an illness or trauma that has caused ear infections that have persisted for more than 3 months, then the chances of developing an auditory processing disorder are higher. Take notice of your child's language and how it is developing. Most importantly, does your toddler understand simple commands, even if you are not looking directly at him?

Perhaps your child has been deaf or partially deaf since birth, and you're just now learning this. This can be heartbreaking news and hard to handle; however, there are many ways to communicate with your child and to help him learn to communicate with the world. Later in the book, we explore music therapy and auditory integration therapy, but there are more programs a specialist will be able to help you with. There are also hearing aids and devices that your pediatrician, audiologist, and/or otologist (ear, nose, and throat physician) will be able to assist you with.

My son underwent speech therapy because I thought that his delays in language were a speech problem, which later turned out to be a hearing problem. Just remember to explore all avenues if your child is having developmental delays. Because the senses are so interrelated, it is sometimes difficult to decipher where the root of the problem lies. It may take a team of specialists working together to determine the best course of therapy for your child. Thankfully, the Individuals with Disabilities Education Act makes these services and evaluations available to all citizens. Talk to your pediatrician and seek out local government agencies to point you in the right direction to getting your child evaluated as early as possible.

Auditory Resources

If your child has a problem with his or her hearing, you can check with these organizations for assistance and guidance: the American Speech-Language-Hearing Association, *www.asha.org;* the Joint Committee of Infant Hearing, *www.jcih.org*; and the National Institute on Deafness and Other Communication Disorders, *www.nidcd.nih.gov/.*

We also recommend these books about auditory processing disorder: *When Listening Comes Alive,* by Paul Madaule, and *When the Brain Can't Hear: Unraveling the Mystery of Auditory Processing Disorder,* by Teri James Bellis, PhD.

How to Find the Help You Need

Always start with your pediatrician. Ask for information on specialists and referrals. Oftentimes, your pediatrician will have pamphlets and information on hand, and his or her network includes specialists of all varieties. Get a second opinion if you are concerned. Your pediatrician will most likely not know you're checking with another physician, and if he does, he will not be offended that you're taking care of your child.

- Visit your local and state government Web sites and start calling around to see what resources are available in your area for children that may have special needs and/or developmental delays. Be persistent. Ask which regional center is your provider.

- Call your insurance carrier and see what is covered. Find out if at least a portion of having your child evaluated is covered.

- Call or visit your local school district's office to see how old your child has to be to be evaluated for their early-intervention programs.

- Attend a local meeting that pertains to your area of concern. Are you worried that your child may have autism? Go to a TACA meeting in your area and ask the other parents where to get started and what to do. Are you curious to see if your child has SPD? Start calling occupational therapy clinics in your area and get your child evaluated.

Not having any luck finding your state's early-intervention resources? Visit Pathways Awareness at *www.pathwaysawareness.org/*. Their parent-answered help line may point you in the right direction with some additional resources, occupational therapists, physical therapists, and organizations.

The worst thing you can do is nothing. Be your child's advocate and seek out the answers and treatments necessary for your child to live his or her best life.

CHAPTER EIGHT

Therapies for the Senses

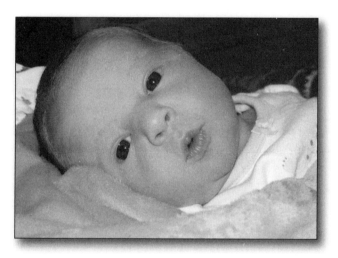

The wonder, hope, and joy of a new baby girl.
ELLISON, 4 DAYS OLD

The Mouth

OUR ORAL-MOTOR SKILLS DEVELOP EVEN WHILE WE ARE STILL IN THE WOMB. You can sometimes even see babies sucking their thumbs on ultrasound images. Babies learn to use their oral-motor skills for the most important skill they require when they are first born—eating! Babies must know how to latch onto a nipple, close their lips appropriately around it to make a seal, and then suck, swallow, and breathe with coordination. Some babies struggle with this task when they are first learning. Sometimes this is due to premature birth, or weak muscle tone, or they may just need practice. Once the baby gets the hang of eating from either the breast or a bottle, she begins to develop stronger oral-motor skills.

As your child gets older and solid foods are introduced, most typically developing babies are able to adapt to rice cereal, veggies, and fruits, and then eventually to regular solid foods. Some babies will go through a stage where they are picky about what they eat and will one day like green beans and the next day spit them out. Keep trying to introduce your baby to a variety of foods so she will have a well-balanced variety of foods she likes.

Refusal of New Textures or Flavors

"My baby is not eating what all my friends' babies are! She tends to gag when she smells certain foods or tastes certain textures." If your baby is beginning to refuse foods, gag, or throw up when presented with new smells or textures, and it's starting to happen more frequently, you will want to contact your pediatrician to see if your child is having any sort of physical problem with swallowing or possibly a sensory issue with food, which could be an oral aversion.

Oral aversions (a reluctance to feed) can be seen in babies as early as birth or show up anytime, when a child begins to refuse foods, gag, or make herself throw up when presented with nonpreferred foods. Some children have such extreme oral aversions that they will gag when you wipe their mouths with a napkin or if they even see a spoon across the room. An oral aversion this intense could mean serious sensory and feeding issues and necessitates a specialist to help address these issues (either a speech-language pathologist or an occupational therapist who specializes in sensory feeding).

If your child has a slight defensiveness to new foods and/or textures:

- At each meal, encourage your child to try something new (from young babies eating baby food to a child of any age).

- Allow her to touch and feel the foods on her plate. It's okay to be messy!

- Encourage other types of media play, like finger-painting, Play-Doh, and sticky or gooey substances (always with supervision and never forced).

- Provide oral stimulation, massage, and stretching, which need to be guided by a speech-language pathologist or occupational therapist.

Oral-Motor Interventions for Hypersensitivity

If your child or toddler is hypersensitive to oral stimulation or defensive to anything in or around her mouth, if she has not been orally fed for a length of time because of medical issues, or if she may be orally sensitive for any other reason, here are some activities you can do.

Use a NUK brush or your finger to gently massage her gums and cheeks, and roll the NUK on her tongue. If she is too defensive for that, massage her gums with a warm washcloth, and allow her to chew and gnaw on the washcloth to get input on her gums and cheeks. Use vibration on the outside of her face and mouth with vibrating teethers, a vibrating toothbrush, or even your own finger and hands "vibrating" her cheeks and the areas above and below her lips. Be careful not to overstimulate your child with vibration, as she may be resistive to this at first. Sometimes, as a therapist, I will even use a toy that provides vibration on a child's cheeks, neck, and shoulders to help desensitize him for when I touch in and around his mouth.

OCCUPATIONAL THERAPIST TIP: For toddlers and preschool-aged children, you can work on oral stimulation during snack time or before a child eats to help stimulate his mouth and then help prepare him to eat. Encourage him to eat crunchy and chewy foods that provide deep pressure to the mouth (proprioceptive input). This can help decrease chewing of other nonfood objects and putting inappropriate things in his mouth.

It is age appropriate for infants to put their hands in their mouths to explore, and they will also put most toys in their mouths to learn about their environment, but this behavior should decrease over time, and toddlers around 2-3 years of age should not be putting everything in their mouths. You have to especially watch that they don't get ahold of small objects that could be choking hazards.

NOTE: Always be careful that you are not sticking things too far in your baby's mouth so that she chokes. Do not leave her unattended with a NUK brush or other objects that could potentially be a choking hazard. Make sure that anything you put in or around her mouth is made for that purpose and is nontoxic.

As your child becomes a toddler, if she's still having oral aversions or an oral aversion arises, try not to argue with her about it. Fighting with your child or forcing her to eat foods will just make an oral aversion worse. You don't want dinnertime to become a form of torture for your child, and it's not going to help to take items away or try to discipline your child for a physical or psychological condition (or a combination of the two). You'll both end up losing.

If your child has more extreme difficulties with feeding, or oral aversion, please seek out a specialist (either an occupational therapist or a speech-language pathologist who specializes in feeding issues). Another good resource is a book, *Just Take a Bite*, by Lori Ernsperger, PhD, and Tania Stegen-Hanson, OTR/L.

Additional Ideas for Feeding Issues

I found myself on a waiting list to have my son work with a feeding specialist. In the meantime, what do you do and how do you feed a child who refuses to eat? Here are a few things that helped me.

First, I was never pushy. I tried all the feeding books and techniques, such as putting food out in ice-cube trays and repeatedly offering it to my son with fewer choices available each time. (Putting food in the trays keeps them separated so they don't touch, and they're little portions for tiny tummies and can hold a variety of choices.) My son would rather have starved, and he would have, had I not extended breast-feeding. He hated textures so much that he wouldn't *touch* any foods, let alone pick them up and put them in his mouth. So what was I to do? I purchased a juicer!

OCCUPATIONAL THERAPIST TIP: Feeding expert and pediatric psychologist Kay Toomey, PhD, who specializes in children with feeding disorders, recently presented at a conference I attended. She says that you should offer a protein source, a fruit or vegetable, and a carbohydrate source at EVERY meal and snack.

- *Juicer.* The juicer was absolutely the best purchase I ever made. Although my son hated the sound of the juicer, I could make carrot apple juice and many other combinations, such as green apple and broccoli, and he LOVED them! I always made sure to put the juices in a dark cup, because if he saw that the color of the liquid was green or orange, he wouldn't drink it. What I learned was that he could tolerate the fine consistency of a juice that didn't have any pulp or chunks in it. I started adding strawberry fish oils to the juice and liquid vitamins, which he drank, as well. The juicer saved my life until we could get my son working with an occupational therapist who specialized in feeding.

- *Health Master.* The Health Master is a massive blender-type object that Montel Williams endorses, which emulsifies food into desserts, drinks, soups, and sauces. Unlike the juicer, the Health Master doesn't rid the fruits and vegetables of pulp and rind—it uses all the contents more like a blender. If your child cannot handle any chunks, then this is not for you. If your child can handle a little more texture, the Health Master is able to make healthy desserts, like homemade ice creams, as well as hot soups. Yum! This may be a way to help you introduce different temperatures of foods while still giving your child a softer consistency that is easier to swallow.

- *Liquid vitamins and supplements.* When your child is not eating, it's terrifying to think that he's either going to starve to death or that he's not getting vital nutrients for brain development. While I know most kids love to chomp on Flintstone vitamins that taste and look like candy, my son wouldn't even let me put the little "Bam Bam" on his lips. I researched vitamins in liquid form that came in a variety of flavors and made sure that they were approved by my pediatrician. We were able to find liquid multivitamins for kids in citrus flavor and fish oils in strawberry flavor. If your child will tolerate it, give it to him in a dropper or medicine spoon. Otherwise, read the instructions or call the manufacturer and see if you can mix the vitamins with juice, applesauce, ketchup, chocolate pudding, or anything else that your child prefers to eat.

- *Straws.* Straws are magical. Use a straw with your child. The sucking is calming because he's having to breathe deeply and focus on the task. He's strengthening his oral-motor skills because it takes a lot of work to squeeze his lips around the straw and use his tongue to suck. Cut the straw in half if he's not able to get the liquid all the way up the straw. Start with easier liquids, like water, and work up to thicker drinks, like smoothies, applesauce, and even pudding.

The Eyes: Light Therapy

Light therapy is a form of treatment that involves exposure to daylight or specific frequencies of light for prescribed amounts of time. It is most commonly used in regions where seasonal affective disorder is prevalent. Although there are still few answers on the effectiveness of bright-light therapy for those that are more severely depressed in cloudy months, some patients have experienced positive results when undergoing the therapy for a number of weeks. Another use of light therapy among adults is alleviating chronic fatigue syndrome.

Occupational therapists, psychologists, and other trained professionals practice light therapy with children who need help regulating and controlling their emotions because it helps build self-esteem, it alleviates balance difficulties and coordination issues, and it helps reduce hyperactivity. There are a number of mesmerizing lighting systems that provide sensory feedback. Many of the lights change color, which is calming in the way that watching fish is relaxing. Oddly, while the lights are calming, they are simultaneously stimulating different parts of the brain and working on a child's visual sense. These therapeutic lights may be used to carry out a variety of tests to assess how much a child can see.

A classic light therapy is to use spaghetti-like fiber-optic lights all around a child, which provides proprioceptive feedback. The child is able to feel where his body is, as if being grounded. Just think if you didn't feel the pull of gravity keeping your feet on the ground—you would feel as though you were floating. For a child who needs proprioceptive feedback, the weight and pressure of the lights around him would feel similar to a ball pit.

Floor-to-ceiling bubble lamps and flat-screen LED lights are known to be calming and have even instigated language production and communication in mostly nonverbal children by means of sign language or computer applications. As always, these are therapies that work differently for each child, and results are not typical.

Light therapy is often combined with auditory stimulation, such as soft music, and touch therapy (such as a massage or maybe feeling a variety of textured beanbags). If you're interested in light therapy for your child (or for yourself), find a multisensory clinic or room within a clinic that provides light therapy in your area to see if this is a therapy you would like to explore further. Start by talking to your occupational therapist or child psychologist to find an expert in your area.

MOM TIP: Use a night-light that changes colors or leaves a pattern of stars on your child's ceiling and walls. This is soothing, and kids love it. Maybe he can help you pick out the night-light when you buy it. This may also help keep your toddler in his room at night!

The Nose: Aromatherapy

Essential Oils: What's All the Fuss About?

Essential oils are most often extracted from plant matter via steam distillation or through pressing. They are not to be confused with perfumes, which have musk or animal products in them, or synthetic fragrance oils that have a different chemical structure and lack the therapeutic benefits of essential oils. What are the therapeutic benefits? There are too many to list, but we'll touch on ones that you will find interesting for you and your family.

Benefits of Essential Oils

It's commonly known that the scent of lavender is calming, which explains why it's used in a ton of baby products these days. However, pure, essential lavender oil has endless benefits, including treating burns, cuts, and stings. It not only stops the pain, it also speeds up the skin's healing process while soothing inflammation. The oils have to be pure, though, or they can cause serious damage to a wound.

Lemon essential oil can help defend the body against infection, and peppermint oil is an antiviral. We're big on peppermint in my house, and I am pleased to report that my son hasn't gotten the flu since starting kindergarten (he's in second grade now) and has made it through the swine-flu outbreak unscathed. It's possible that the peppermint oil we use to calm his stomach is a factor. Eucalyptus oil may be used in a diffuser if your little one has a cold. This oil acts as a decongestant, with very powerful antiviral properties. Tea tree oil can be used for fungal infections, blisters, cold sores, and insect bites.

Interestingly enough, essential oils are used topically to aid the skin, as well as on pressure points to promote relaxation. They can be diffused into the air to benefit everyone in the room. One suggestion is to put a few drops of an oil of your preference onto a cotton ball and put it by a vent in your room. You will enjoy the benefits of fresher-smelling air without having to use candles or chemical air fresheners.

Essential Oils Meet Western Medicine

Thanks to the American Holistic Nursing Association and similar organizations, aromatherapy is being used in hospitals and doctor's offices across America. Nurses are using essential oils derived from herbs, plants, and seeds to aid in pain management for patients with cancer and to help treat anxiety and depression, and, most commonly, Alzheimer disease. As recent as January 13, 2010, *The Medical News* published an article titled, "Olfactory Dysfunction May Serve as an Early Diagnosing Tool for Alzheimer's Disease." We can no longer ignore our sense of smell as unimportant and regard it as a luxury to sniff the roses when we get a chance, instead of recognizing it as a vital emotional receptor. The nose is important business.

"The sense of smell is the only one of the five senses directly linked to the limbic lobe of the brain, the emotional control center. Anxiety, depression, fear, anger, and joy all emanate from this region," says D. Gary Young, ND, in his book, *Essential Oils, Integrative Medical Guide,* published in November 2006.[16] Young also states that "because the limbic system is directly connected to those parts of the brain that control heart rate, blood pressure, breathing, memory, stress levels, and hormone balance, essential oils can have profound physiological and psychological effects."

Aromatherapy has become a staple in the spa and massage industry, and estheticians may use essential oils while giving facials. Chiropractors, physicians, neurologists, and occupational therapists are becoming certified in the science of adding clinical aromatherapy safely into their practices. We recommend that you become certified in essential oils before practicing with them and talk to your physician before even thinking about experimenting with essential oils. There are many professionals out there to advise you and guide you to a positive essential-oil aromatherapy experience.

Suggested Reading

We recommend the following books about aromatherapy and essential oils: *Aromatherapy for the Healthy Child,* by Valerie Ann Worwood, *Essential Oils Integrative Medical Guide,* by D. Gary Young, ND, and *The Complete Book of Essential Oils & Aromatherapy,* by Valerie Ann Worwood.

Music Therapy

"Children in general, who are having difficulties, and especially those with disabilities, are typically not heard. If a child knows, consciously and unconsciously, that they are truly being listened to, you would be amazed how easily they become motivated and deeply engaged."

—ANDY TUBMAN

Interview with Music Therapist Andy Tubman

Music therapist Andy Tubman has had a busy year. He has traveled to India twice to speak to doctors, therapists, and teachers about "music and the brain" and autism. He's presented in Nashville on the benefits of music therapy, as well as at the San Gabriel Regional center, where he is a vendor. I was privileged enough to sit down and pick Andy Tubman's musical brain, and what I found was both inspiring and fascinating. First things first, Andy does not teach children how to play musical instruments, unless he believes a therapeutic goal can be attained through the process. Music therapy is far more complex and visceral, depending more on a therapist's intuition and ability to connect with a child to get the desired results.

- *Why music therapy?*

  Since parents are always going after therapies and treatments with scientifically based results, I asked Andy why a parent would choose music therapy for his or her child. He pointed out that one cannot argue with the increase in electric activity in the brain that music therapy stimulates. An example can be found in nonverbal children and/or children on the autism spectrum, who often have an underdeveloped Broca area of the brain (which pertains to the process of understanding language and gestures and the release of audible language). These children may demonstrate a notable improvement in language and communication skills after undergoing music therapy. Musicians have highly developed Broca areas. In other words, music therapy may be able to improve a person's ability to communicate. Sound cool? It gets even better.

- *A Typical Music-Therapy Session*

  The therapy is entirely dependent on the child and what he or she gravitates to. Andy sets the room up in terms of "creating stations." If the child is interested in drawing, Andy may strum his guitar and sing to the child while he draws. He reflects what the child is doing verbally with the lyrics of the song. Musically, the energy and the tempo of the music are designed to be a reflection of the child's behavior and movement. As long as the child accepts Andy's song, the child is unknowingly receiving a variety of therapeutic benefits simultaneously. The music Andy provides is helping to "structure" the activity, while the child is encouraged to express himself and increasingly contribute to the music as the session progresses. Communication and speech, taking turns, awareness of self and others, attention span, developing creative coping strategies to deal with feelings of overwhelm, response time, vocalization, and the ability to communicate needs are all enhanced with music therapy.

Andy uses the ISO principle, which involves musically matching the energy level of the child he is working with. If the child is angry and has his arms crossed, Andy will play something with some energy to it, in a minor key. That way the sound of the music will closely reflect the child's mood and energy. (Kind of like when you're sad, you typically listen to a sad song.) During a breakup, you might listen to Sinead O'Connor's "Nothing Compares to You." Andy believes that if you can match a person's energy level, then she will be more likely to follow the therapist in facilitating music that leads to another energy level or another mood.

One student that Andy works with, Gavin (names have been changed for privacy purposes), has glutaric aciduria type 1, a disorder in which the body is unable to break down certain amino acids. This causes his body to stiffen painfully, amongst other ailments. As a reaction to his frustration, Gavin was taking out his rage by kicking his mother. Andy created a structure musically that matched his energy and frustration level. He started singing a song, in which he said, "You can kick the drum." Gavin kicked the drum. By doing so, he began working out his aggression, understanding the message lyrically, making music, and also working on his deeply impaired gross-motor movement control (an added benefit). As the boy's anger started to subside, Andy added more to the song: "Kick the drum...not your mom," to which Gavin laughed, and his energy transformed into that of a happier child. Gavin no longer kicks his mom. Since he was responding positively to music therapy with Andy, he was able to start undergoing sensory biofeedback sessions in combination with music therapy to help him regulate his breathing, increase his oxygenation, and soften his musculature. It seems the more I learn about music therapy, the more I understand the far-reaching extent of its benefits.

Andy uses a variety of instruments during therapy, which may include percussion instruments, drums, piano, and an array of guitars. He also uses supplies that kids are familiar with and enjoy, such as clay, paints, and colored pencils, and he customizes the sessions to accommodate the specific needs of the patient.

"As the child's interests open up, typically so does her desire to improvise and make music," he says. "When I support children in making music and I'm really stimulating the brain universally in positive ways, that's when you start to see serious changes in speech and behavior. In music, the rabbit hole is endless as to how deep and complex it can go."

- *Benefits of Music Therapy*

Andy sometimes works with children with behavioral problems. He gives them a safe outlet that is typically structured within a musical context. He has screamed with them within a song if that's what they need, but notes that a therapist has to be careful during this type of an intervention, so as not to reinforce a negative behavior. It's a fine line and a very subtle difference in knowing when you're helping to soften a behavior or starting to reinforce one, but he listens to his clients on multiple levels and observes their body language.

Clients come to him for a variety of reasons, but many are looking to increase their children's attention spans, help them to be able to express their needs, improve their communication skills, work on pronunciation, and help them regulate their bodies and calm themselves.

- *Do Parents Participate in Music Therapy?*

The process starts with a full assessment and evaluation of the child, with the parents' involvement (aka filling out lots of forms, which us parents of special-needs kids are used to doing on a daily basis!). Andy then talks to the parents about what their goals are for their child and what they would like him or her to work on. For the next month, Andy gets to know the child during therapy, and then he presents the parents with long-term and short-term goals, which are broken down into increments.

Andy then teaches the parents how to help the child self-regulate or be musically supportive at the right stage in the child's therapy. Once the child is ready, he encourages and begins to teach the parents how to either dance with their child or perhaps drum with their child during a session. Since the parent spends the most amount of time with the child, it can be beneficial to integrate the parents into specific sections of the therapy to follow through at home in between therapy sessions. At that point, the sessions can become a form of family therapy, as all parties benefit. The idea is to have the parents help the child utilize the benefits of music outside of a therapy session, when needed, and to keep the child's relationship with music a healthy and positive one.

When asked what he thinks about finding the right kind of therapist for a child, he recommends that parents find one that really knows how to connect with their child—a difficult task, since a new therapist has not typically been observed in action. Andy may offer the parents of his clients a video of a typical Integrative Music Therapy session or have them remain in the therapy room until everyone is comfortable.

- *Principles and Theories behind Andy's Practice*

Andy has studied multiple principles, including those of A. S. Neill and Nordoff-Robbins, and through his own experiences as a music therapist, he has created Integrative Music Therapy. As he works with many children with autism, Andy uses music as a bridge between our external world and the children's internal worlds. If the child is deeply engaged, or having fun, and is interested in the therapy and what he is doing, then it is easier for Andy to achieve the desired results and goals.

The theories behind his practice coincide with much of what Britt and I preach: Provide structure and support for the child in a nonrestrictive environment, allow the therapy be led by what the child gravitates to, and never force a child if he's not comfortable. Andy's mission is to help unlock creativity, provide paths of communication, build confidence, and support physical and mental health and overall well-being.

- *How Andy Became a Music Therapist*

  Andy Tubman was led into music therapy by a traumatic event that happened early in his life. Shortly after high school, his best friend had a car accident and flew through the windshield. He ended up in the brain-trauma unit. Andy would sneak into the hospital and play the guitar for his friend. He only knew a few Elvis songs, and he admits that he wasn't a particularly strong player, but he played and sang nonetheless. His friend underwent a series of surgeries and remained in a coma in the intensive-care unit for a couple of months. Andy continued to play for his friend, who awakened from the coma, mouthing the words of a Pink Floyd song Andy was playing. There were many witnesses in the room at the time, and a nurse suggested that Andy talk to the music therapist at the hospital. The next semester, he enrolled in the music-therapy program at Temple University in Pennsylvania.

  Upon graduation, Andy completed an internship at Norristown State Psychiatric Hospital, where he learned firsthand about life in an institution. His first job as a music therapist was working at a school for children with severe behavioral issues, which was run by an adjacent psychiatric hospital. Since then, he has fine-tuned his music-therapy skills with a wide range of psychiatric patients, from children to the elderly.

- *Andy's Current Projects*

  Andy Tubman cofounded U-Sing, a technology-based music-therapy intervention, for which he ran a research project at the prestigious Beth Abraham Family of Health Services, known for being the home of Oliver Sacks *(Musicophilia* and *Awakenings).* Andy's music therapy company, Integrative Music Therapy Services, or IMTS, can currently be found serving the communities of the "West Side" of Los Angeles (Cornerstone Music Conservatory), Alhambra and Roland Heights (with the Chinese Parents Association for the Disabled), and Malibu (at Echo Malibu, a teen-recovery treatment program). To contact Andy, please visit his Web site at *www.integrativemusictherapyla.com* or e-mail him at *andytubmanimts@gmail.com.*

The Ears

Auditory Integration Training Interview with Khymberleigh Herwill-Levin

- *What Is Auditory Integration Training?*

Auditory Integration Training, or AIT, is the most powerful intervention that a parent of a special-needs child can consider. It's a painless, noninvasive, drug-free, and amazing solution that can deliver results in less than 2 weeks. Auditory Integration Training is a safe, effective sound-based training that efficiently retrains a disorganized auditory system and improves processing distortions and sound sensitivity. Berard AIT has been proven highly successful for children with autism, sound-processing disorder, learning disabilities, and special needs, as well as for typically developing children and adults. Berard AIT is an educational intervention that was developed by Dr Guy Berard and is based on a scientific protocol that is backed by more than 30 years of scientific research.

- *Method and Results*

Approved candidates listen through headphones to modulated music from an approved AIT device twice a day for 10 consecutive days. This provides each individual with a total of 10 hours of listening training, completed in 20 30-minute sessions. An approved AIT device and a specific type of music must be used, and the protocol must be followed to ensure the desired results.

Some of the results that parents, teachers, and therapists have reported include improvements in awareness, responsiveness, expressive and receptive language, interest in communication, articulation and voice intensity, auditory comprehension, better attention, focus, and memory, as well as a reduction in distractibility, inappropriate behavior or stimming, impulsivity, and antisocial behavior. These are just a few changes that could be brought about—there are so many more, from improvements in bed-wetting to eating, sleeping, and developing balance for riding a bike, dancing, playing sports, and making music.

The human body is continually being influenced by internal and external sound stimulation and vibrational activity. Each organ in the human body responds to a different sound frequency. When the auditory process is not working properly, it can interfere with our entire physical system and our overall health. Our ability to function in harmony will be affected. The way our bodies respond to and process sound activity affects us intensely and differently. Sound (and the frequency of sound) affects our overall health, mood, energy level, alertness, attention span, focus, concentration, information processing, and the way we express ourselves, both verbally and in writing.

Once the cause of the auditory processing problem is corrected, all therapy and other educational interventions can often become more effective. Changes can then occur that enable the client to achieve at a greater level.

- *What age groups do you work with?*

I have worked with all age groups, from 3 years old to 76 years old, all with extremely good success. If I am working with a child who has received a diagnosis of a particular disorder, the younger she begins to do AIT, the better the results (early intervention is key).

- *What do you do if a child won't wear the earphones?*

I have been doing Berard AIT since 1994. During this period, I have only encountered three children with whom I have had to struggle for the full 20 sessions to keep the headphones on. Most children resist for the first 2 days. This is understandable, since they do not know me and are not really sure what I intend to do with them. Once they realize that this unique training is not intrusive or painful, they adjust and often enjoy the rest of the sessions. I always warn parents that the first 2 or 3 days are the hardest, that I am firm but very kind and gentle. I am the one that makes sure the headphones stay on the child's head.

- *What types of music do you have to choose from?*

The music that all certified Berard trainers use has been approved for use and covers a wide range of frequencies. Most contemporary music covers only a narrow range of frequencies, often between 750 Hz and 3,000 Hz. We try to use a larger range, often between 125 Hz and 8,000 Hz. It is also important that the music source has ample tone and a vigorous beat. In general, music considered acceptable for AIT includes reggae, rock 'n roll, pop, and jazz. I generally start my young clients with children's music. This calms them down and makes the sessions more comfortable and enjoyable. Most classical music is not appropriate for AIT. The need for varied frequency and a fast tempo come from Dr Guy Berard's clinical experience.

There are no current scientific studies that support the importance of these recommendations.

- *How did you learn about AIT, and when did you start practicing?*

In 1989, my eldest son was diagnosed with an auditory processing disorder and a severe learning disability. We were told to do all the conventional therapies that were available to us. We saw a little improvement, but considering the time he was spending at therapy sessions, the improvements were diminutive.

There were not many resources in South Africa in those days, where we were living, but I was directed to a wonderful doctor who diagnosed my son's condition in a matter of a few hours. (He received a diagnosis of pervasive developmental delay, not otherwise specified). She then suggested doing AIT, which we arranged soon after. Within the next 6 months, both his teachers and I observed extensive changes in him, both scholastically and behaviorally. I remember how, before we did AIT, his third-grade teacher commented to him, "You seem so happy in your world—tell me where you are, I would love to join you." After AIT, she stated that he was very aware, focused, and extremely connected with his surroundings. His behavior improved, and he started doing much better at school.

After I had learned about the benefits of AIT, I began to understand why, after doing all the conventional therapies we are taught in college, some children still did not improve, or their improvements were slight. I then realized that if your auditory system was not operating correctly, then how could you expect your whole neurological system to operate accurately?

In 1994, I decided to study further and train to become an AIT practitioner. (At the time, I had an MA in special education.) I opened my first clinic in Cape Town, South Africa, in 1996. Since then, I have traveled around the world, from Africa to Israel to the United States, working with many children and adults who have experienced tremendous benefits from doing AIT.

- *Is there anything else you'd like to share about AIT?*

I'd like to share my bio (which was not written by me) from my Web site, so your readers can learn more about me and how passionate I am about AIT:

Each and every day, Khymberleigh Herwill-Levin becomes an advocate for children with special needs! Through her company, "Learning to Listen/The Brain Fitness Center," more than 4,000 children have seen positive, significant changes in their lives. In the past 14 years, parents from around the world have sought out Khymberleigh's assessments and treatment for their children. They have placed their trust in her to provide outstanding, professional services that improve their children's abilities. The methods she employs are proven, safe, and highly effective for not only children, but also teens, young adults, and adults. The comprehensive assessment creates the basis of her treatment plan for her clients.

Khymberleigh personally tracks the progress of those enrolled in AIT. With her professional follow-up, all the components of the treatment program are drawn together for the benefit of each client. As a professional consultant and a hands-on practitioner, you can be assured of the highest-quality care and specific results for your child or yourself.

Khymberleigh now resides in both California and Nevada with her five beautiful children. She is dedicated and is extremely passionate about her work.

KHYMBERLEIGH HERWILL-LEVIN
Learning to Listen/The Brain Fitness Center
PO Box 1557
Zephyr Cove, NV 89448
www.ait1st.com

The Skin: Baby Massage

While massage has been around since the dawn of time and is practiced regularly in other cultures, it's only now becoming more mainstream in the United States. We all know that massages work wonders on a stressed, fatigued, and sore body, but what are the benefits for an infant and child? Besides being another way for a parent to bond with her child through touch and eye contact, it is also wonderful for tactile stimulation and proprioceptive awareness.

As the sense of touch is accessed through the skin, the millions of touch receptors in the skin send signals to the brain constantly—there is no "off" switch. Whether your baby is awake or sleeping, eating or playing, happy or upset, she is always receiving these tactile messages. A warm touch from a parent's hand on a child's body may trigger the release of oxytocin, a hormone that stimulates a sensation of trust and aids in reducing the stress hormone known as *cortisol*. Most often, massage will make your baby very relaxed, but there are times when your baby is wide awake and wants to play. At this time, massage may be more stimulating and cause your baby to be more alert. Pick an appropriate time to massage the baby, such as before an afternoon nap, and not right after he wakes up and is eager to explore. Some experts say that massage enhances growth and development, promotes communication, and enhances neurological development. It is also used by trained professionals to help relieve a baby's discomfort and to encourage healing in the NICU.

It is highly recommended that you take an infant-massage class before practicing massage on your newborn, especially if your baby is a preemie or has medical concerns. There are chains like Liddle Kidz that have pediatric massage-therapy certification programs throughout the U.S. and Canada that instruct you on the proper and most effective ways to massage an infant and toddler. They also offer a program designed for massaging children on the autism spectrum and have found that massage may aid in relaxation and could reduce some behavioral difficulties. Being that massage is basically a form of sensory integration and works well along with an occupational therapist's daily sensory diet (on an individual basis), then it should be noted that massage may help decrease aversion to touch. Some parents have said that massage has helped their children with sleep issues, as well.

Massaging different areas of the body will aid your baby or toddler in different ways. If she has gas or a stomachache, massage can help her get relief. If your baby is cranky and tired, the methodical movements may soothe her into a more relaxed state.

There are many wonderful nontoxic massage oils available to make your hands move effortlessly across your baby's skin, and the scents can promote even deeper relaxation. Plus, your hands are moisturized, and by giving a massage, you're getting proprioceptive input, too! Try not to use too much oil, as your baby is tiny, and you don't want to lay her in the crib afterward and get oil everywhere. Also, oil on your hands and on your baby's body will make your baby slippery. Keep a baby blanket close by to wrap her up in before carrying her to the next destination or before putting her into the bath. Make sure that the oil does not get into the baby's mouth, nose, eyes, or ears![17]

Acupressure

We talked to acupuncturist Emily Calvanese to educate ourselves about the ancient Chinese practice of acupressure. Here is what we uncovered. For more information on acupuncture or acupressure, please talk to your primary-care physician or your child's pediatrician for a referral.

- *What is acupressure?*

  Acupressure means applying pressure to specific acupuncture points (there are no needles!). In Chinese medicine, there are 12 primary and eight extra channels that span the length of our bodies. Along these channels are points, each with a specific indication and purpose. So we can press on certain points (or use needles to access them in acupuncture) on the basis of what is going on healthwise with the child or adult.

- *What acupressure points can be beneficial to help calm your baby or toddler?*

  There are many points that can be extremely beneficial in terms of calming your baby or toddler. Typically, babies and toddlers really enjoy acupressure and find it very calming and relaxing. It is very soothing and is great to do right before bed or naptime. When finding points, it is helpful to note that measurements are taken according to the patient's individual body. When working with a child, you want to use his finger or hand width as a guide in the following descriptions.

  The following is for informational purposes only, and must be administered by a trained professional.

  Gentle but firm pressure should be used. Some points that are easy to find and very helpful include:[18]

  - Ki 1, which is on the bottom of the foot, approximately on the midline, one third of the way from the base of the toes to the heel, about one finger-width from the end of the ball of the foot.

- ST 36, on the lower leg. It is one finger-width lateral to or outside of the shin, or front edge of the tibia. It is one hand-width, measured at the knuckles, below the bottom edge of the kneecap, or patella.

- Sp 6, also on the lower leg. It is on the inside of the leg and measures one hand-width above or proximal to the medial malleolus or inside anklebone.

- LI 11, on the arm at the elbow crease. If you bend your child's elbow, it will be at the outside or radial end of the crease.

- LI 4, on the top or dorsal side of the hand. It is between the thumb and forefinger.

- Yin tang, between the eyebrows. It is in line with the inner corners of the eyebrows and is right in between the two.

Each point can be pressed on for a few seconds at a time, using your thumb or index finger. Points don't need to be pressed on in any specific order, and both sides don't need to be held at the same time. Again, use gentle but firm pressure.

You can also press gently along the sides of the spine, using a line that is halfway between the child's spine and medial edge of her scapula or shoulder blade. Follow this line from the crests of the shoulders to the base of the spine with that same gentle pressing movement, pressing every half-inch to 1 inch. This opens up the energy flow in the child's back and is very relaxing.

NOTE: It is important to note that these points serve as guidelines, but it would be advised to contact a licensed acupuncturist in your area for treatment. Many of these points should be avoided by women who are pregnant or by children or adults with certain health issues.

- *What acupressure points can be beneficial to help calm a stressed mother or father?*

  The same points and massage listed above would be helpful to calm a stressed parent. In addition, you can try pressing on:

  - LV 3, on the top of the foot, between the big toe and the second toe. It's about halfway back from the base of the toes to the spot where the first and second metatarsal bones meet.
  - GB 21, on the crests of the shoulders, halfway between the spine and the edge of the shoulder.

About Acupuncturist Emily Calvanese

Emily Calvanese obtained her master's degree in acupuncture and Chinese medicine from Oregon College of Oriental Medicine in Portland, Oregon, and is currently practicing at Acupuncture Northwest. She continues to be inspired by watching how well Chinese medicine works in treating children. In her practice, she treats adults and children, which gives her the wonderful opportunity to see, treat, and learn from all ages. She works with a wide variety of disorders, including pain, digestive disorders, women's health issues, asthma, allergies, insomnia, nightmares/terrors, depression, anxiety, stress, learning disorders, attention-deficit disorder, ADHD, and sensory-integration disorders. Emily lives in Portland with her husband and 3-year-old son. They love spending sunny days outside, exploring the Pacific Northwest.

CHAPTER NINE

Environmental Factors

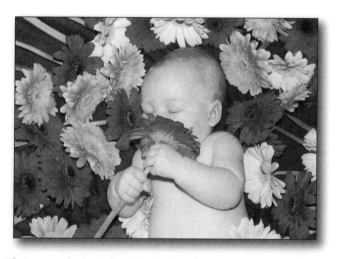

*I have to admit, I glued a Gerber daisy to my son's diaper
and it stuck to his stomach! I felt like the worst mother ever.*

ODIN (JACKIE'S BABY), 2 MONTHS OLD

Toxins in Your Home

MANY PEOPLE ARE "GOING GREEN" THESE DAYS, AND AS KERMIT THE FROG
said, "It's not easy being green." As a society, we're doing what we can,
but it is impossible to completely remove toxins from our world, as they're
in everything. We are not trying to scare you—it's scary enough to be a
parent! However, we would like you to be aware. While we cannot rid

our world of toxins, we are constantly adapting and changing as information becomes more available. Britt and I no longer use Styrofoam food containers, and we have switched to stainless-steel water bottles instead of plastic. If we do use plastic, it's BPA free. As we learn, we adapt. Following are a few ways to make positive changes for your sensory health—especially your baby's sensory health. Studies have shown that chemicals and toxins affect children more than adults because they're still developing.

Cosmetics and Toiletries

Thankfully, there are more environmentally friendly options to "paint your face" (as my mom used to call applying makeup). As a parent, start reading labels and go for the brands that use natural and organic contents. I was appalled when I read about the dangers of hair spray, as I grew up on lethal doses of Aqua Net. According to Kirkman Kleen's Web site and catalogs, where you can find a complete list of toxins in products and their related effects, hair spray may contain chemicals known to be toxic to the central nervous system and kidneys, as well as cause developmental defects in boys' genitals. No more hair spray for me! After reading about the toxins in everyday products on that Web site, I threw out all the cosmetics and products in my bathroom. I now only use products that are made with fewer chemicals and more natural elements. Interestingly enough, I'm often saving more money by using nontoxic chemicals rather than spending more, like I thought I would have to.

Another example of a cosmetic product that has been linked to cancer, amongst other diseases, is nail polish. Again, I went on a search for nontoxic options for nail polish and nail polish remover. They exist! Nontoxic nail polish, made without formaldehyde, is available at your local Whole Foods or online at *gonatural.com.* I tried it out, and it works the same as toxic nail polish and costs the same amount. The nontoxic nail polish remover admittedly stinks, but the toxic kind has a distinct odor, as well—we're just used to it.

National Allergy Supply provides lines of nontoxic shampoos, soaps, sunscreens, and other products that we recommend. They're mostly fragrance free and leave you feeling clean. If you're looking for a yummy fragrance, Origins is a brand that creates everything from natural deodorants to makeup, as well as products for men. Burt's Bees is another popular brand that uses natural ingredients with pleasing results. Tom's of Maine is dedicated to healthy dental care. Their toothpaste, mouthwash, and floss are made without any toxic colorants, scents, or preservatives, and they all receive the American Dental Association's Seal of Acceptance. Apparently all those chemicals are not needed for a clean mouth—imagine that! The more popular these nontoxic products become, the more pressure competitors will feel to remove their dangerous chemicals, as well.

There are numerous nontoxic choices for your baby. A new eco-friendly baby cosmetic line pops up every day, and we welcome them. It was upsetting to me that when my son started speaking, he told me he hated the Elmo bubble bath I had been using for years. He explained it made him itch and hurt his bottom.

Studies are showing that talcum powder can irritate your baby's lungs, ears, eyes, nose, and throat, so think twice before exposing your baby. Use nontoxic cleaners when washing the baby's pacifier or binky. When you wash your baby's hands, use a nontoxic soap or nontoxic hand sanitizer. Just say no to baby chemicals! Remember, new moms, your baby cannot tell you how she feels, so please use the products that won't cause your baby physical irritation and harm.

Cleaning Products

If you watch Oprah, Dr Oz, or any number of science and discovery shows, you have probably seen how toxic household cleaners can be. Instead of going into the million reasons as to why you should not use these, we will instead provide nontoxic options for you.

- *Carpets and rugs.* Recently, we had a guest who got food poisoning, and let's just say, she didn't make it to the restroom a few times. It was even worse than a pet accident! After using our trusty steam cleaner with a nontoxic carpet cleaner, an odor remained in the room. I read online that using baking soda on dry carpets worked, so I tried it. After sprinkling the baking soda on the floor all around the room and leaving it overnight, my room spelled fresh and clean without using any abrasive lethal cleaners. Keep babies and toddlers away from baking powder, though, as you don't want them to inhale it.

It's recommended to use baking soda to absorb greasy stains overnight, but don't try to clean it up while it's wet, as it will just get clumpy and crystallize, making it harder to vacuum up. Another good tip is to use an ice cube to harden gum or remove candle wax (this also works on human hair) and to use a household item such as club soda to remove the dreaded red wine stain after a holiday meal.

- *Kitchens, bathrooms, and laundry rooms.* Okay, so who enjoys cleaning the bathroom? I don't, especially because I live with my husband and son! Boys do far more damage to a toilet than girls, or at least *my* boys do. Here are some nontoxic solutions that will get you through your sanitizing duties.

  While you can make your own cleaning products by finding a number of recipes on the Internet or in eco-friendly books, there are nontoxic brands at most stores that sell cleaning products. Seventh Generation, Simple Green, and KD Gold are product lines that are effective and have generally nonirritating smells. Even though your windows, counters, and floors will shine, you may have to listen to your in-laws complain that it's not truly clean unless it reeks of Formula 409. It can be difficult to teach older generations new and environmentally friendly ways, but even they will probably grow to appreciate the less offensive cleaning smells in time.

  White vinegar is pretty impressive. My front-loading washing machine developed a mold problem in the rubber casing around the door. I ran the self-cleaning cycle on the machine and then scrubbed the rubber with white vinegar, and it removed the mold. I now get to clean the rubber regularly and keep the washer door open when not in use to ensure that it stays dry, but at least the harmful mold is at bay. Vinegar one, mold zero.

- *Laundry and linens.* Brands such as Seventh Generation offer a variety of fabric cleaners and softeners. Your clothes will come out just as clean as the old-fashioned products we were raised on. If you live in an area where weather permits, hang your clothes and sheets out to try. The sun acts as a natural disinfectant.

Plants—More Than Just Pretty Green Things

It's a good idea to go green, literally, and add a few potted plants to your living space.

A study by Dr Bill Wolverton has shown that some houseplants can clear carbon dioxide and volatile organic compounds from indoor air. Which plants are most effective? The Boston fern removed the most formaldehyde, and the peace lily worked best on acetone. For more amazing information on which plants are good to keep in your home, see the book, *How to Grow Fresh Air: 50 Houseplants That Purify Your Home or Office.* The only thing you have to be wary of is if a plant is poisonous if eaten. Do not keep poisonous plants in your home for any reason. It's not worth it for you or your baby.

Additional Toxins in the Home

If you or someone in your home is sick or has an illness, one factor to consider is the toxins you already have in your home. Talk to your doctor about testing your drinking water (as well as the water you shower in, as toxins may enter your body through your skin). Perhaps you should test for lead in your paint, pipes, and water. Is there asbestos in your insulation or vinyl flooring? Many houses are known to have mold, some of which is extremely toxic and detrimental to one's health. There are a number of kits you can use to test your home yourself, or you can hire a professional mold tester in your local area. Could there be arsenic in your hardwood floors?

Since it can be hard to pinpoint where the poisons could be coming from, consider hiring an environmental assessor to do all the work for you. These can be found on your state government's Web site, under "toxic substance control," or you can call an environmental nonprofit agency in your area for a recommendation. I, for one, wouldn't know how to evaluate local power lines and the voltage I may be receiving. An environmental assessor should be able to notify you of the amount of toxins in your home and in your area.

A Personal Example from Jackie

Both my son and husband had severe allergies and had been pre-scribed daily allergy medication. It was suggested that we put a dehumidifier in the house to help keep mold and moisture at bay. While the dehumidifier helped, my son's allergies kept getting worse. His eyes were irritated and watery with dark circles under them, and he had a constant nasal drip that caused a chronic cough. It was frustrating to use a medication to battle an obviously environmental toxin, so we scoured the house for the source. We found hints of mold in his walk-in closet, deep in the back, behind a row of clothes. Upon peeling away the paint, we found layers and layers of mold that had been painted over! Since we were renting, instead of going through an entire rebuild, we moved, and my son is no longer having to take allergy medication. The mold seemed to be causing all of his symptoms, from birth to 3 years old. Never once did my pediatrician or allergist suggest that I test my home for toxins. I hope they do now that I shared my story with them. I'm sure countless others who have uncovered pollutants in their homes are having similar positive health results, as well.

Tox Town

As we all know, like germs, toxins are everywhere. While there are too many to list in this book, we found an amazing Web site brought to you by the National Library of Medicine, called Tox Town, found at *tox-town.nlm.nih.gov/index.php*. In Tox Town, you may click on a variety of areas, including restaurants, hair salons, the beach, a farm, and more, and it will show you what toxins are lurking and how to avoid them. It's a fascinating Web site, and it points out safety concerns, as well as toxins. The site is also available in Spanish.

Suggested Reading

If this is a topic of interest to you, and since we have only scratched the surface, here are some books that further explore toxins and their effects on babies and children. There are also a number of informational Web sites to help guide you as you adopt a "green" lifestyle. We recommend *Healthy Child, Healthy World: Creating a Cleaner, Greener, Safer Home,* by Christopher Gavin, *Raising Healthy Children in a Toxic World,* by Phillip Landrigan, and *Raising Baby Green: The Earth Friendly Guide to Pregnancy, Childbirth, and Baby Care,* by Alan R. Greene.

Diet

Diet crazes change with the wind in this country. Something is good for you one day and bad for you the next. Everyone is searching for a magical pill to cure all ailments and make us skinny, but is that even possible? Probably not. We all know that when a woman is pregnant, what goes into her body goes right into the baby's body via the placenta, and then through her breast milk if she breastfeeds. But what do we feed our babies once they are ready for solids? How do we know which fruits and vegetables are safe from pesticides? How can we tell if our baby has a lethal peanut allergy or an intolerance to gluten? What foods are best for our babies and families? Like anything else in this world, there is no one answer.

As you make food choices for your family, remember that everything that goes into our bodies affects our moods and behavior, as well as our brain development and our ability to function. Have you ever noticed that you felt lethargic after a big Thanksgiving meal? Or, worse, have you ever gotten a headache or felt fuzzy headed one day because you ate only carbohydrates and starches? Is your child often violent, or does she have a behavioral outburst a few hours after she eats? Does your baby rub her eyes and get a runny nose after eating certain foods? Monitor your child's behavior and see how quickly you notice mood changes after she eats or if she complains of not feeling good afterward. Does she get really hyper and then crash? Does she get tired suddenly? Is she able to sit and focus or is she jittery and agitated?

Food and Your Child's Mood

Neurotransmitters (brain chemicals that affect how we think and feel) are composed of the building blocks of protein and choline, which are obtained from our diet.[19] Anger, anxiety, depression, fatigue, impulsiveness, and distractible disorders are all being linked to food intake and nutritional deficiencies. You want to ensure that your child has the proper nutrition for her brain to continue to develop and thrive, as well to encourage physical and emotional development. Elizabeth Somer, MS, RD, author of *Food & Mood,* explains that every day, you are building your child's food associations and memories, as well as her emotional cues that urge her to eat and to crave certain foods, which will shape her food preferences.[20] While that may seem like a lot of pressure and difficult to figure out in the day and age of massive marketing campaigns, the easiest way to figure out what is good to feed your child is by monitoring her moods, behavior, mental clarity, and ability to function after eating. Feed her the foods that work best for her body, and feed yourself the ones that work best for yours.

Sensory Eating

Food is sensory—when you eat, you experience the way it looks, the way it smells, the way it tastes, and the texture. If your child doesn't like the way her toast is cut, or her peanut butter is too chunky for her, or perhaps the plumbing is backed up and the kitchen smells rancid, your child's eating experience can turn into a negative one. Are her legs stuck to the plastic high chair? Is her diaper dirty? Is the restaurant you're in too noisy and hectic for her to concentrate? On top of being a personal chef, it's important to create a positive sensory atmosphere for your child to have a successful eating experience.

On a more scientific level, neurotransmitters are constantly conveying information to the brain and nerve cells about our environment. These chemical messengers translate many sensory messages, such as if we are hot or cold. Neurotransmitters are affected by the foods we put into our bodies. Help regulate your child's neurotransmitters by feeding her healthy foods daily.

Most of the time, children are fairly easy to feed and will adapt to different environments, but be considerate of your child's sensory needs during mealtime and help her to develop lifelong healthy eating patterns.

Addictions, Cravings, and Habits

Research has proven that our bodies become addicted to certain foods, causing us to crave them. Unlike pregnancy cravings, addictions usually occur with bread, pizza, bagels, ice cream, and carbohydrates made of wheat and dairy products. People who crave carbohydrates may have an imbalance of serotonin.[21] What does that mean? Well, serotonin is a neurotransmitter that regulates intestinal movements, mood, appetite, sleep, muscle contraction, and cognitive functions such as memory and learning. Pharmaceutical companies synthetically control serotonin levels with antidepressants and antianxiety pills, such as Prozac.

Sometimes we eat for emotional reasons, like the old cliché of how a woman eats ice cream after a breakup (I know I'm guilty!). Sometimes we're not hungry, but we eat out of habit, because it's "time to eat" or because we're at a weekly social event or because we're just used to eating a bag of chips while watching M.A.S.H. reruns late at night. Pay attention to when you're eating and why. You may be surprised at what you discover about yourself and your eating patterns, and how this affects your physical well-being.

As a parent, you are responsible for what your child eats. If he is underweight or overweight, it is due to either medical causes or what you are feeding him, or both. Your kids eat what you eat and what you buy and are only as healthy as you allow them to be. Setting your child up for a successful relationship with food is in your hands.

Marketing Campaigns

Just because you are bombarded by commercials, print ads, and public service announcements about how product is "healthy" or "good for you" does not mean that it is! The açai berry has arrived and is being strongly pushed by diet pill manufacturers as an antioxidant. Soy products have been expending a seemingly endless marketing budget over the last decade; however, some people have an adverse reaction to the estrogen-high bean (no matter what form it's processed into). Those multimillion-dollar celebrity ads with "Got milk?" mustaches are gorgeous! Who doesn't want those slim figures, which are practically guaranteed if you drink tall glasses of liquid gold every day? Well, my son, for one, who is lactose intolerant. Milk does not do his body good, but it does for others, and that's okay. Try not to be smitten by these campaigns and so-called promises, and do your own research on what food products are best for your body and your family. Now, if I could just figure out how to look like Paris Hilton in a bathing suit while eating an enormous, juicy burger.

Food and Your Body

The best way to tell if your nutritional needs are being met is by paying attention to how you feel. Are you stressed out? Constipated? Tired all the time? Hungry all the time? Cranky in the afternoons? Do you have severe PMS? All of these are symptoms of not eating the right foods for YOUR body. Just as you monitor your kids' reactions to what they eat, take note of your own reactions to food, as well. If you have concerns about your diet or that of your child, there are many nutritionists and food experts to consult with. Another person to check in with may be your psychologist, if you're concerned you may have an eating disorder. Food and emotions go hand in hand, and it may take an expert to help get you on track. Best of luck, and happy eating!

Baby Food

What is in baby food? Mostly fruits and vegetables, but it is worth it to seek out the brands that don't add sugar, food coloring, and preservatives. As we've mentioned before, your baby is more susceptible to toxins than you are, so feeding him the least-processed foods is important, as they are easiest on a baby's digestive and sensory systems while he's absorbing vital nutrients. For amounts to feed your baby and information about storing baby food, please talk to your pediatrician and follow manufacturer instructions.

Fruits and Vegetables

To be or not to be organic? As a girl who was raised in a farming community, I used to think that organic food was a bunch of marketing nonsense, but as more and more research has come out about the health benefits of organic produce, I've now converted to the organic side. With organic fruits and vegetables, there are still some pesticides and fertilizers, but the fruits and vegetables cannot be genetically modified if they are to receive the organic label. Often, organic fruits and vegetables are more expensive, but more and more grocery chains are becoming organic friendly and more competitive, since consumers are wising up and making healthier choices for their families. We get enough food additives and chemicals from everyday foods and products, so it makes sense to limit the toxic intake of our most nutritional resources. Organic fruits and vegetables may not *look* as healthy as genetically modified fruits and vegetables, because there are no red dyes in the tomatoes or growth hormones added to the broccoli.

If you buy in bulk at stores such as Costco, which I do often, you can find fruits and vegetables that haven't been pumped with chemicals. Also, washing your produce upon getting home can remove some of the harmful pesticides. If you're bringing home canned food, check for additional sugars, such as fructose or corn syrup, as well as additives and preservatives.

MOM TIP: Frozen fruits can be a delicious dessert, either blended into a cold smoothie or partially thawed in a bowl. Make sure no sugars are added to these naturally sweet treats! Purchase bags of frozen berries and mixed fruits, or make your own by cutting up pieces of your child's favorites into kid-friendly pieces. You can even make your own popsicles out of pureed fruit. Yum!

Kids and Caffeine

Caffeine is one of those tricky chemicals that children react differently to. You may be familiar with caffeine sometimes being used to calm children who are hyperactive, and yet caffeine makes other children bonkers. According to Jack Challem, author of *The Food-Mood Solution,* caffeine increases the secretion of adrenaline and cortisol (the "stress" hormone), while decreasing levels of calming neurotransmitters, such as serotonin and gamma–aminobutyric acid, or GABA.[22]

Caffeine is a stimulant and is found in chocolate, sodas, coffee, and energy drinks. Some kids build a tolerance to caffeine, while others grow agitated, experience withdrawal when they do not have it, and experience negative effects to their sleep cycles. Make sure your child drinks lots of water when he ingests caffeine, as caffeine has been known to dehydrate.

Kids and Protein

Knowing that protein is the primary source of nutrients for neurotransmitters, it's highly recommended that you talk to your pediatrician and/or pediatric nutritionist to ensure that your child is receiving proper amounts of protein. As one size doesn't fit all, you need to research the best sources of protein for your child, taking into consideration possible food sensitivities, allergies, and intolerances. While some kids do well with meat, such as chicken, others respond better to sources such as peanut butter or cheese.

MOM TIP: Broccoli is usually a pretty safe choice for protein. If you're having a hard time getting broccoli into your child's diet, try blending it up with green apples to make a juice or a soup— it's delicious!

Salt

What is salt? It's sodium and chloride. Salt has been implicated as a factor in insomnia, air and motion sickness, and Meniere syndrome (an agonizing ear ringing).[23] Sometimes we crave salty foods, like potato chips or ham, and this could mean that you are dehydrated, as salt encourages you to drink water and fluids. Other times, salt causes you to bloat and hold onto liquids. Salt is in almost every food, including the pancakes you ate for breakfast, the bread on your sandwich, and the soup you ate at lunch, as well as the meatloaf and mashed potatoes you had for dinner. Get the picture? We eat a lot of salt without thinking about it. Watch how much extra salt you're putting on your meal for taste, and try other spices and alternatives if you're seeking flavor.

Sugar

Many people, including doctors and scientists, have said that the idea that sugar makes a child hyper is a myth. Just as many doctors and scientists say it is not a myth. So what's the answer? How can it NOT affect your body? Anything that goes into your mouth or your baby's mouth affects your chemical makeup, the nutrients in your body, the amount of insulin that is produced, your digestive system, your nervous system, and so on. Everyone reacts differently to different substances; however, kids have smaller bodies than we do, and what they intake is processed faster than it is in adults.

Glucose is known to lead to bursts of energy and rapid mood swings, hunger, irritability, and physical weakness.[24] Be wary of junk foods, treats, cereals, and products that may cause your child to have an overload of glucose, which will in turn mess with your child's natural insulin production and distribution.

More often than not, you and your child are going to eat some sugar throughout your day because it is in most foods; however, try to keep it to a minimum and be aware of how much you are consuming. While sugar is tasty, it's not necessarily good for our growing brains and waistlines. A cookie here and there will not hurt you, unless you don't feel good afterward or your child has an adverse reaction to the cupcake he ate.

The different names of sugar on labels include sugar, brown sugar, glucose, fructose, lactose, maltose, sucrose, corn syrup, high-fructose corn syrup, and maltodextrin, amongst others.

Food Allergies and Intolerances

Food Allergies

Food allergies are on the rise, and parents should take note if their child seems to be having a negative reaction to one or more food groups. What should you be looking for? Common signs of a food allergy are hives or a rash on the skin, itchiness and/or swelling of the tongue or throat, shortness of breath, wheezing, stomach pain, vomiting, and diarrhea.

Milk and soy allergies can show up at birth, if milk and soy are used to feed a newborn. Since you will most likely be taking your baby to a doctor (or possibly an emergency room) if any of these symptoms occur, then food allergies will be one of the many things that your pediatrician will look for. Skin tests and elimination diets are the most popular forms of testing for food allergens with children. Depending on how severe the allergy is, some children will be able to have small amounts of the food they're allergic to, and some allergies are so severe that they are lethal.

These allergies are more likely to occur in families where the parents have allergies, as well, even if they're not food allergies. If both you and the baby's father have allergies, then be sure to start a food-allergy journal as your baby starts eating more and more foods.

We talked to one mom about her experience with a daughter with severe food allergies. This is what she had to say.

- *How did you first know your daughter had a food allergy? What were the signs?*

It was clear to us within the first few months of life. She started to develop rashes (eczema) on her face and behind her knees and in the creases of her inner arms. The rashes on her cheeks were bright red and irritated. We consulted with our pediatrician, and she recommended that we test for food allergies and also referred us to a pediatric dermatologist. The tests confirmed many food and environmental allergies, which led to asthma appearing about 2 years later.

- *What are some of the changes you've had to make as a mom and as a family to live with food allergies?*

Our lives changed instantly. Our daughter is allergic to eggs (even cooked within foods), peanuts, nuts, seeds (all types), and a variety of other foods. This changed how we shop at the grocery store, what we can cook for meals, and how we approach traveling, holidays, school, and every aspect of life. We learned to read labels and find foods that don't contain the allergens we have to avoid. Our whole family subscribes to the same diet, and we don't allow any of the allergens into our home. We don't eat out at restaurants, and we have to enlist the help of friends and family at social gatherings. Food allergies have affected our lives on a daily basis.

We also learned that our daughter had many environmental allergies, such as trees, grass, mold, dogs, and cats. These environmental allergies seemed to worsen her asthma. Unfortunately, this can make many things difficult, like outdoor sports, playing outside, campfires, going to homes with pets, and many other things. We've learned to figure out what her "triggers" are and to avoid those things as best we can. Otherwise, we have learned which medications can help and how to use them when necessary.

- *Have you noticed any other sensory sensitivity with your daughter?*

Yes. Our daughter has always been sensitive in various ways. As a little girl, and even today, as an 8-year-old, she is sensitive. One of the more noticeable things has been her aversion to certain clothing and particularly tags in her clothing. This was really a challenge for a long time. She objected to wearing any clothes with tags. She also wouldn't wear clothes with a "waistband" of any sort, so it took years and years to get her to agree to wear jeans. She's never liked socks and generally complains about things being uncomfortable! She tends to wear clothes she likes over and over again. These things seem to be less of a problem now than it was a few years ago.

- *What would you like people to know about raising a child with food allergies?*

Raising a child with food allergies is really a struggle every single day. Food is something that becomes a major decision at every turn. Most people don't have to think about food to the extent that we do and can just eat what they want, wherever they want to! For us, we have to work hard to find recipes and meals that don't contain allergens and cook from scratch a lot more. When our daughter is invited to a birthday party, we need to send a safe cupcake or cake along with her, because she can't have whatever the other kids are having. When we go out trick-or-treating, we pay her for the candy she can't have (which is just about all of it!). Most of all, our daughter has learned that sometimes (okay, many times), the answer is just "No, you can't eat that." I think that has been the most painful part of the experience—watching your child miss out, knowing that she is missing out, and feeling helpless to change it. With food allergies, you have to accept what you cannot have and learn to live without it. I know some people think that parents of children with food allergies are just overreacting, and that is hard. I would never choose this for my child, and I wish people knew how hard it is and how we'd do anything to not have this daily challenge.

Food Intolerances

Food intolerances are not food allergies. *Intolerance* is defined as either a hypersensitivity to a food or the inability to digest a food because of a lack of enzyme or stomach chemicals to break down the food properly. Intolerances can go unrecognized and untreated for years and may also develop or worsen over the years. The most common food intolerance is to milk products, because of the lack of the enzyme lactose.

Signs of Intolerance

Physical signs of intolerance may include sinus congestion or chronic congestion, bloating, diarrhea and constipation, dark circles under the eyes, night sweats, poor balance, headaches, skin rashes or canker sores, swelling of the hands and/or feet, coughing and sneezing, muscle spasms, and cramps.

More cognitive, emotional, and behavioral signs of food intolerance may include hyperactivity, tantrums, insomnia, lethargy, depression, anxiety, and the inability to focus or think clearly.[25]

If you feel you or your child might have an intolerance to food, try the elimination diet. Only remove that one item or food group from your diet for a time period, and see if you notice a substantial difference. Kenneth Bock, MD, author of *Healing the New Childhood Epidemics Autism, ADHD, Asthma, and Allergies,* recommends removing casein (milk products) for 3 weeks and removing gluten (wheat products) for up to 3 months to see what differences occur in a child's symptoms. Work with your pediatrician to put together the best team of experts and specialists for your child. They will be able to guide you and uncover the best nutritional plan for him.

Jackie's Experience with Food Intolerances

I disagree with the term "abnormal" when it comes to food intolerances. Why is it abnormal for our bodies to be intolerant to different foods? Isn't it possible that those foods are not good for most of us, if any of us? With the onset of rampant disease and obesity, maybe—just maybe!— processed foods made with wheat and dairy aren't good for us. Obesity, celiac disease, diabetes, Crohn disease, and autism diets all recommend removing gluten and dairy to heal the gut and uncloud the brain. Dr Atkins, who is well known for his extreme protein diets, originally started the diet for his heart patients, who needed to unclog their arteries and get their blood pumping more freely. He therefore removed gluten and dairy from their diets. All of the diseases I've mentioned here are connected to food. It's something to think about.

I took the advice outlined previously on food intolerances, and I stopped giving my son milk products for more than 3 weeks. After 2 weeks, his teacher called me and asked what I had done, because he was able to focus and stay in his chair during lessons. She said that his anxiety had decreased, and he was participating with the other children more—and that was just from removing milk! We were so excited, we cleaned out the entire pantry and refrigerator, dumping anything and everything with gluten and casein, additives, food coloring, and soy. We got rid of it all. I have to admit that our cupboards were bare, until we made a trip to Whole Foods to load up and develop a new way of eating. It has truly been a lifestyle change for the entire family.

Now, when my son has gluten at a class pizza party or cake at a friend's birthday, everyone comments on how he's "out of control," "off the charts," and "like they've never seen him." I use those rare occasions to validate my lifestyle change and am thankful that we finally figured out that food was causing many of his behavioral and physical disabilities. He's progressing by leaps and bounds, and everyone in the family is benefiting. I've lost those extra pounds off my waist, and my husband has more energy. I know we're in the low percentage of people who are intolerant to gluten and casein, but it's working for us, and we're feeling healthy and happy.

One company I can recommend for gluten-free, casein-free, and soy-free foods is NuLife Foods. If needed, they can also provide foods without corn, shellfish, eggs, milk, peanuts, soybeans, tree nuts, and wheat. The customer can choose whatever they want, on the basis of their own lifestyle needs. The chicken nuggets are "to die for," and they have meatballs, pancakes, and a wide assortment of foods to choose from. The totally wonderful thing is that their food tastes like REAL food and is actually delicious enough that you could serve it to guests, and they wouldn't know it was a restricted-diet food! For more information, you can locate them at *www.nulifefoods.com.*

CHAPTER TEN

Medical Concerns

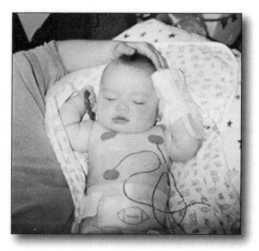

*While it can be scary to have your baby in the hospital,
it's comforting to know they're in the best hands.*

RYAN, (JULIE'S SON), 8 MONTHS OLD

Preemies

WAS YOUR CHILD BORN PREMATURELY? IF SO, CHANCES ARE YOUR BABY HAS already been seen by a neonatologist in the NICU and hopefully an occupational therapist, physical therapist, and/or speech-language pathologist who specializes in working in the NICU.

When your baby is born premature, there are other precautions and things you have to take into consideration, depending on your baby's needs. A lot of babies that are born early have difficulty with breathing on their own, delayed motor skills, and difficulty feeding (coordinating their suck-swallow-breathe reflex), among other medical struggles. Many premature infants need special machines to help them breathe, lights, and warmers, among other medical necessities. A team of doctors, nurses, and therapists will attend to them around the clock.

Occupational therapists and physical therapists can help organize your infant's sensory systems to help him be able to feed, sleep, transition, and tolerate touch. Speech-language pathologists can also help by working with the physical needs of eating and swallowing safely.

When you have a child that has been born early, you really need to pay attention to his developmental milestones to make sure that he is meeting them, even if he is behind. Hopefully, he will eventually begin to catch up. It is so important to work on things like tummy time, visual stimulation (but not overstimulation), oral stimulation (to make sure she is latching well and feeding efficiently), and developmental play skills, and to watch for any signs of medical issues. Many programs around the country follow preemies by means of a developmental clinic that tests babies at certain ages, such as at 3, 6, 12, 18, and 24 months, to make sure that the babies are developing at a healthy pace.

Many premature babies will need occupational therapy to address their sensory needs, play skills, and motor skills, amongst other things. The earlier you can start the appropriate therapies for your premature child, the better. Premature infants who are born really early (23-29 weeks) are at a greater risk for having cerebral palsy. Most doctors are going to watch your child closely for signs of cerebral palsy, but advocate for your child, make sure you are taking all necessary precautions, and do your research.

Premature babies are often subject to extended hospital stays, which can be hard on the new parents. We talked to an expert, Yamile C. Jackson, PhD, PE, PMP, about her experience with her preemie son and loving inspiration, Zachary, and the company that evolved from her experience, Zakeez, Inc. As an occupational therapist and mom team, we find her story and products to be an incredible asset to other parents who are in her situation.

- *Yamile, what was your experience with Zachary being born prematurely?*

In 2001, I gave birth to my son, Zachary, 12 weeks prematurely. He was born to save my life, because I had severe preeclampsia. He weighed less than 2 pounds, and when he was 3 weeks old, tropical storm Allison hit Houston, shutting down power to the hospital. The hospital staff and my husband and I had to keep Zachary alive by hand for 9 hours, until he was evacuated. It was at that time that I made a promise to do whatever I could to help all babies—and I prayed for the opportunity to do it on Zachary's behalf, not in his memory. The 155 nights Zachary spent in the NICU were like riding a roller coaster (and not a good one!). He experienced the flooding after the storm, a lot of pain, several surgeries, and a number of other unpleasant experiences— even a projection of life of only 6 months to 2 years—and he held on.

I have always been aware that we learn about and comprehend the world through our senses, and all he was sensing of the world was pain and suffering (except when I could hold him). I didn't need the PhD in engineering to know that he was experiencing gravity too soon, and that it had to be very difficult for him to move. I knew that there had to be a better way to teach the babies to move without so much stress and without losing energy that they needed to grow.

I spent at least 10 hours a day with him, and I hated leaving him at night. It was not enough to know that I loved him—*I wanted Zachary to know that I loved him,* and I couldn't do that if I was not present. I also learned from the nurses how to use my hands to comfort him—how to hold him and how to touch him to give him boundaries. Often, I told my husband, "I wish I could cut off my hand and leave it with Zachary," because I wanted something to continue to comfort Zachary in my absence. I sewed hand-shaped pillows, which I slept with so that they would pick up my scent (and my husband did too!), which I could leave with Zachary to keep him feeling loved, warm, and secure when I couldn't be there.

The nurses showed me the difference in Zachary's monitors when the "hands" were cradling him, especially if they were scented by me or by my husband. Seeing that he was at ease helped me feel more relaxed, my separation anxiety and sense of impotence eased, and my breast-milk supply increased. Two weeks after I finally brought Zachary home, I received a call from the development director at the NICU to see if I could make her "little hands" for the other premature babies, and I knew this was how I could keep my promise to help babies and their parents.

- *Has your son had sensory issues and/or dysfunctions?*

Soon after Zachary was born, one of the first questions that I asked the nurse was, "What is a common denominator of preemie babies when they grow up?" She said, "Babies in the NICU usually grow up not liking to be touched or hugged." I also heard, "Preemies have a difficult time bonding with their parents." This was the first "sensory issue" that I tackled consciously. I believe that touching is an expression of love. It is a bonding experience, and I find it very comforting. Kids run to their parents when they hurt, just for a loving touch, which helps them feel better. When we are sad, a touch to the shoulder makes us feel better. There is nothing better than a loving hug. Touch connects us. *I could not imagine giving my son a life without the ability to enjoy human touch.*

I spent 10 hours a day in the NICU, and I touched Zachary and held him, skin-to-skin, for at least 5 hours a day, which I now know is not enough. When I wasn't holding him, I ALWAYS left my scent on his hands pillow, or "Zaky," 24/7.

After we came home, I noticed that I could not restrain his movement (such as in a tight hug), because he did not like it. We worked for a couple of months to teach him that not all restraining of movement was going to be followed by the pain of a medical procedure, and then I could hug him so hard! Later on, he was bothered by clothing tags and had some textural problems with certain foods, but both were resolved soon, with the help of the occupational therapists.

- *In what environment did your son work with occupational therapists?*

Zachary's occupational therapists worked with him at the NICU and then at home for about 2 years. We would not have had the success story we did without competent professionals. I believe what made a difference was that the therapists took the time to teach me not only what I needed to do, but what signs to look for, and what to expect. It was very beneficial to have experts guiding me the entire way and working together as a team to get him well. Now Zachary is a healthy and smart boy, thanks to the team of professionals that worked with us and the support of our friends and family.

- *As a result of your experience, you created the "Zaky," the bonding, therapeutic, and positioning pillow, ergonomically designed to help the baby feel comfortable and protected while assisting parents and their children feel closer to each other. What are the sensory benefits of the Zaky and the Kangaroo Zak?*

The idea of our two products is to give premature babies 24/7 contact with their parents and to also promote stimulation, relaxation, sleep, and growth. Ideally, the parent holds the baby, skin-to-skin, with the Kangaroo Zak as long as possible, and when they are not holding him, then the Zaky provides support, stimulation, and a sense of security.

Both the Zaky and the Kangaroo Zak provide touch and relaxation, so the baby spends his energy growing and not looking for boundaries. With the Kangaroo Zak, the baby not only feels the skin of the mother or father, but the parent provides ideal and permanent thermoregulation. With the Kangaroo Zak, the baby is in an environment as close to the womb as possible, which provides containment and minimizes stressful movement. The Zaky minimizes the association of touch with pain, which I believe is what makes the NICU babies terrified of being touched. With the Zaky, the baby receives a soothing touch that is sometimes combined with warmth and the scent of mom and dad.

With both products, the baby has the smell of his parents nearby, which is very important to his well-being. Additionally, when the baby is inside the Kangaroo Zak, he is close to the heartbeat, the breathing, and the voice of his mother, just as he would be inside the womb. Once the baby comes home from the hospital, he can listen to the sounds of the environment and acquaint himself with the voices of his family members and the noises of the house, while in a very safe location (against the chest of his parent). Although the kangaroo position limits his field of vision, he can see face of his mother and/or father.

All of these factors represent the benefit of getting to know the world (in which the baby arrives abruptly) through the security of contact with his mother. This also empowers the mother, as she gets to know her child and is able to stimulate him and give him the security to face external stimuli. Our products also help parents by decreasing separation anxiety and a sense of impotence, while fostering the bonding process and a sense of control and empowerment.

- *How did the Zaky come to fruition?*

I made a career change—I went from being an engineering management consultant to spending the next 3 years developing the Zaky. I used my PhD in ergonomics and human-factors engineering and my personal experience to refine the original hand-sewn design, and I researched and tested it until we brought the Zaky to market in 2004. I have spent the past 3 years researching kangaroo mother care and designing the Kangaroo Zak, which I wished I had when I had Zachary. Both products are now available in many retail and online stores and are used in hospitals nationwide. They have won a dozen awards. Zachary is now our CIO (Chief Inspirational Officer) of Zakeez, Inc, and we have a program called "On Behalf Of Zachary," or OBOZ, to donate our products to sick babies around the world.

For more information about Yamile C. Jackson, PhD, PE, PMP, and the Zaky, please visit zakeez.com.

Hospital Stays

Hospital stays can be sensory disasters. Not only are you stressed out and worried about your child and all the medical unknowns, but hospitals are not designed to be accommodating to your sensory systems. What if your child has a medical condition that requires several hospital stays and possibly surgeries? How do you make the hospital your home away from home? We talked to one mom, Julie Neininger, whose baby, Ryan, was diagnosed with Hirschsprung disease, a form of bowel obstruction. Ryan ended up having several surgeries to remove sections of his colon and intestine. He also underwent colostomies, which is when the intestines are connected to a bag for bowel discharge. Sound stressful? It was. Here is how Julie dealt with the sensory overload and emotional stress of hospital procedures on her son's road to recovery.

• *How did you find out about Ryan's condition?*

Ryan was nursing fine after birth. Then, after circumcision, he wasn't nursing much and didn't want to nurse. They sent us home from the hospital anyway, even though he hadn't passed all the meconium (the first stools), which we now know is an indicator of Hirschsprung disease. We went home for a couple of hours. Ryan wasn't nursing, and he wasn't crying. Looking back, I guess he was lethargic. We called the hospital a few times and finally went back. I wanted to go right back to the maternity wing, and not an ER. First they treated it like a lactation problem, even though I knew it wasn't. They admitted him and started doing all kinds of tests to rule out everything. That's when his Hirschsprung disease was diagnosed. We spent the next 12 days in the hospital, and he had surgery on day 10. We were sent home two days later.

We continued to have hospital stays for additional procedures— we spent about 5 days in the hospital for the big surgeries and 2 or

3 days for most of the other things. We became regulars for the first few years of Ryan's life.

- *What were the hospital stays like, from a sensory standpoint?*

Sleeping was usually a problem. The hospital wanted him to sleep in a crib, which looked like a cage. I never liked to put him in it, because I never left him alone, and he didn't sleep in a cage—I mean crib—at home. We practiced attachment parenting, where he slept with us at home, and I wasn't about to let him sleep away from me at the hospital. I usually slept in the chair in the hospital room. The sides and arms were big that so I could put Ryan next to me, and we could sleep safely. During the first couple of years, I had to sign a waiver. Then they did away with the waiver, and it was a big problem every time! They were persistent in what they wanted, but as a mother, so was I. In the end, it was always ultimately my child and my choice, and I never gave up what I believed was best for my child to comply with their rules.

The hospital was not very comfortable. People came in all the time, and I didn't get much sleep. The doctor's rounds started very early. Nurses and interns often came in to take vitals. I finally got to where I would ask them to come back later, if Ryan was asleep, and if it wasn't necessary! Mike, my husband, usually brought me food. I typically took a shower when he was there, or I'd run home to shower and come back. It really drove me crazy that there was never a clock in the room. I don't know why they didn't have clocks.

We were there quite a bit, and the hospital staff got to know us. They tried to give us our own room whenever they could. They were usually bright rooms with a window (which was nice), and the hospital was old, but clean enough. There were little TVs that were right by the bed, so that noise wasn't too bad between rooms. I didn't have to hear anyone else's TV. The monitors that Ryan was hooked up to were not too bad, or maybe you just get used to them. Or maybe knowing that they're keeping your child alive makes the beeping okay.

I don't know how you prepare yourself for your child's surgery. I'm not sure how I did it, and it never gets easier. You don't really have a choice, you just do it. I guess I learned as much as I could about what was going to be done and then tried to stay with him as long as possible. It was best if they gave him some medicine to make him sleepy before they took him from us. If the medicine started working before they took him away, it was less traumatic for all of us!

In general, the staff was friendly, and they grew to love Ryan, they just didn't like that I wouldn't put him in the crib—they had their rules! We usually brought toys and books and taped pictures and Ryan's artwork on the wall to make the room more sensory friendly for him during his stays.

- *What advice would you offer to parents if their child is faced with a hospital stay?*

  My advice to parents going through similar situations is to do what you feel is best for your child and make the hospital your home away from home!"

We also talked to Crystal Santos, mother of Alexander, about her extended hospital stays. Crystal's baby was born in San Diego and was later moved to Los Angeles.

- *What was your experience with Alexander like?*

  Alex was born at 37 weeks, and he had a milk allergy, in addition to a blocked intestine. We had to stay in the hospital for almost 3 months, off and on. It was a terrible experience and a shock, when you are so ready to celebrate having this new little person in your life. We were fortunate that the surgeon made room for his surgery to be done when he was 2 days old. Your thoughts daily are, "This is not what I signed up for."

  We were not able to stay with Alexander in the NICU in the first hospital. It was excruciating to leave my newborn nightly. Thank God for the room and care we received at the Ronald McDonald House, so that I could be across the street from the hospital. Many of the women who just gave birth had a hard time being extricated and separated from their new babies, who needed them more than ever. The set-up was horrible! When we moved to the pediatric intensive-care unit and the other units in the hospital, I was allowed to stay, and that gave me more comfort. When we transferred to Cedars Sinai, it was amazing, and we had our own room. I never needed to leave Alex.

- *What was the sensory environment like for you and Alex in the hospital?*

It was busy and noisy in the NICU, except for during certain hours; however, I was happy about it because Alex sleeps through everything and is very scheduled. At the first hospital we stayed in, the lighting was fluorescent. It was cold in the hospital, and I always wore sweaters. It was often loud, with the hustle and bustle of the staff coming in and out and doing what they needed to do. The monitoring machines were pretty loud, albeit necessary. Our room always smelled like disinfectant, but at least I knew it was clean!

At Cedars Sinai, we had a much different experience. They made sure that noise was kept to a minimum, the lights were not bright, and the temperature was ideal. When they cleaned, it did not smell like disinfectant, and they cleaned thoroughly, every day. The cleaning staff asked us if it was okay to come in, to make sure they didn't disturb Alex. Each room had its own temperature controls. It was great!

- *Now that your son is home and doing fantastic, what would you tell moms who are going through what you did when he was born?*

You really have to hang in there. And be aware that you are your child's advocate. Places like our first hospital are understaffed and super busy. Crucial things sometimes get overlooked. Never, never, never leave your child alone, when possible! You could miss a doctor or an important activity, or something crucial can be overlooked in your child's care when you are not there. I know this firsthand. You are only human, so it's hard to be vigilant by your child's bedside.

Let a grandparent or spouse take a turn, but never, never, never leave your child alone. Remember there are also many people that come into the room and care for him or her, and sometimes they are not aware what the others have or have not done. Not to mention, it is scary for a child to have so many new people flitting in and out. They need the security of familiar people. If you are worried, speak up—it can make a huge difference. Also, bring a laptop with you, and look up things you are told at *www.webmd.com.* Ask the nurses for any literature on a potential diagnosis (they are happy to help).

I will say that I felt very secure in leaving Alex for a few moments at Cedars Sinai—they were well organized and kept the same team in place at all times. We did not experience the hustle and bustle of many new people in and out of the room there. They even try to maintain the same nurses. There were no rotating doctors or nurses, and each person was well informed. We experienced no mistakes or mismanagement in Alexander's care. The doctors also came in at the same time every day. Cedars Sinai really gave me peace of mind, and I was able to step away and get something to eat without having a panic attack. They were super attentive to him as a baby and to his special medical needs. Also, they did not release Alex until he was 100% ready to go home and start his healthy new life. Overcrowding and understaffing in other hospitals can get your child pushed out before he is ready to go...I experienced this, myself. It is detrimental to the child's overall health, and you end up right back where you started. This is when you have to become your child's biggest advocate. Fight for him or her. If you feel something is wrong, chances are, you are right!

Cerebral Palsy, Hypotonia, Mental Retardation, and Seizures

Cerebral Palsy

Cerebral palsy is the inability to control motor function. It manifests as decreased coordination abilities and is usually diagnosed within the first 6 months of life. It is sometimes diagnosed at birth. Cerebral palsy can range from very mild to severe. As a therapist, I have seen children with a diagnosis of cerebral palsy, and you cannot even tell. They may have slightly decreased coordination on one side and wear a foot brace, or have one hand that is slightly weaker than the other. They could also have a typically developing brain and cognitive level, but their physical body is delayed. Some children with cerebral palsy are in wheelchairs. In more severe cases, a child may not be able to take care of herself and is completely dependent on a caretaker.

Children with cerebral palsy benefit from multiple types of therapy, depending on their needs, which include occupational therapy, physical therapy, and speech therapy. Physical therapists can help them with walking, leg strength, balance, fitting braces for their feet and ankles, if needed, and wheelchair fitting. Occupational therapists will work on play skills, developmental milestones, core strengthening, self-feeding, dressing, grooming, writing or using adaptive communication devices, and more. Speech-language pathologists work on language development, understanding of language, feeding skills, communication devices, and more. If your child has been diagnosed with cerebral palsy, you need to research the diagnosis and possible therapies and treatments that can be helpful to your child. After assigning a diagnosis, most doctors will help set you up with the correct resources.

OCCUPATIONAL THERAPIST TIP: Always remember that when conducting research on the Internet, make sure the Web sites you view are valid and written by physicians and experts. Take information that you get from the Internet with a grain of salt and know that every child is different, so just because one mom's blog says that her child needs one thing, it does not necessarily mean it will fit the needs of your child.

Hypotonia

Hypotonia is decreased muscle tone and can be caused by trauma, genetics, and central nervous system disorders such as cerebral palsy, Down syndrome, and muscular dystrophy. Usually the cause is unknown. Babies with hypotonia are typically called "floppy babies" because they have poor muscle tone, and their limbs tend to be loose and floppy. Usually muscle weakness occurs because of the poor muscle tone, necessitating physical and occupational therapy to help increase muscular strength. Children with hypotonia can have difficulty eating and swallowing and require specific occupational therapy or speech-language pathology treatment, as these difficulties can be a safety risk due to choking and/or aspiration. (Aspiration is when food enters the airway after swallowing.)

Mental Retardation

Mental retardation is the most common of developmental disabilities.[26] For a child to be diagnosed with mental retardation, she has be tested by a developmental pediatrician or a psychologist to test her in various areas, such as intelligence (IQ) testing, adaptive skills, and developmental living skills. Mental retardation can vary from severe to mild, or even borderline. Children with mild mental retardation tend to have IQ's between 55 and 70. These children are still able to live full lives, marry, hold down jobs, and interact socially with their peers. Children with moderate mental retardation tend to have IQ scores between 40 and 55. They require more assistance to function in their everyday lives and have more difficulty interacting within society. Children with severe mental retardation have IQ scores between 25 and 40 and require extensive support but can usually learn some way to communicate.[27]

Many times, mental retardation can coexist with other disabilities, like Down syndrome, autism, and genetic disorders. Other times, a child can have increased cognitive abilities but have other delays.

Seizures

Seizure disorders can range from infantile seizures to epilepsy. "A seizure may be defined as a temporary, involuntary change of consciousness, behavior, motor activity, sensation, or automatic functioning."[28] Individuals are considered to have epilepsy if they have recurring seizures. Seizures can be a scary thing, especially if you have never seen or experienced someone having a seizure episode. If your child is having what is called a generalized tonic-clonic seizure (grand mal), she may fall to the ground, stop breathing, or experience a loss of consciousness, a loss of bowel and bladder control, and contracting or convulsing muscles. If your child is having an absence seizure (petit mal), she may show signs of loss of consciousness, but this could be so brief that you don't even catch it. Children who have this type of seizure usually stay in one position and look as if they are staring off into space. They may also blink rapidly. Infantile spasms typically begin at 6 months and disappear around 24 months, but they can be detrimental to a child's development, since this is a crucial age of motor and cognitive development.[29]

There is that old saying, "Laughter is the best medicine," and we believe that to be true. As someone who works in the hospital environment, I know that all children, no matter how sick they are, enjoy a good laugh (make sure it's not painful for them!) or a nice smile.

Epilogue

As we conclude this book, we hope that you have learned a lot about your child's development and the opportunities to help your child grow up with a well-balanced sensory system. We also hope that you have learned more about how to utilize your parenting skills effectively for the optimum benefit of your child. We know everyone makes mistakes, and luckily, our children are resilient and can bounce back. Learning to care for your child is an experience that can be both wonderful and frustrating, but we hope that our book has made some of the steps a little easier, and maybe you have learned something about your own sensory systems that can help you understand how your child's systems work.

As our children grow, there are many more sensory developments to explore. In our upcoming book series, we will give tips and suggestions on keeping your child's senses healthy as she enters elementary school, becomes a friend, starts organized sports or cub scouts, and continues to be a sensory being. We will tell you how to keep your child's sensory systems intact and how to keep up with the latest trends, therapies, and environmental discoveries. Games and learning are an important part of childhood, so we'll be writing about which types are best for your child's senses and brain development. It's never too late to start becoming more aware of your own senses and those of your family members.

Thank you for being a part of *Sensory Parenting!*

— Britt and Jackie

Appendix A

Parent Survey

WE ASKED 200 PARENTS FROM ACROSS THE UNITED STATES THE FOLLOWING questions via *surveymonkey.com* (a Web site that tracks your computer's IP address, so you may only answer each survey once). It was interesting to find out how parents are raising their babies and to learn the information they wish they would have known and would like to pass on to other parents. Thank you for sharing your parenting experiences with us! We celebrate you and all you do. Most importantly, we wanted to give you a voice if there was anything you wanted to share to help other parents—and we feel you have. THANK YOU!

NOTE: To conduct the survey, we posted the link on Facebook group pages (parenting groups, autism groups, sensory groups, special-needs groups, single-parent groups, military family groups, etc), as well as on our Web site and a couple of other places. We know some of the parents, but most were folks we didn't know, who volunteered to fill out the survey on the Web.

How many weeks were you pregnant?

Overdue – more than 40 weeks 28.0%
Right on time – 40 weeks 36.5%
38-39 weeks 25.0%
36-37 weeks 9.4%
34-35 weeks 0%
32-33 weeks 2.1%
Even earlier than that! 2.1%

Are you aware of your baby's sensory needs?

Yes, completely 100% 50.0%
Not really, I don't feel sensory needs are important 0%
Somewhere in between choices A and B 38.3%
I have no idea what sensory needs are or
    how to tell what they are 12.8%

Does your baby/child have any sensory sensitivities?

Eyes 3.2%
Ears 36.8%
Nose 7.4%
Touch 15.8%
Taste 14.7%
No sensitivities 56.8%

More specifically – sensory sensitivities include:
Loud noises, vestibular, external stimuli such as excitement over friends/
company/events, sort of aware of textures when feeding/touching food,
balance, muscle tone, core strength, perception.

How often does your baby sleep?

24/7, anytime, anywhere 18.2%
Most of the night, waking for feeding; naps throughout the day 62.1%
Four to 5 hours a night, plus several naps through the day 4.5%
What is sleep? My baby must be a robot! 15.2%

Boob or bottle?

Boob...39.6%
Bottle...20.8%
Both...39.6%

Does your baby use a pacifier or "binky"?

Yes...20.2%
No...46.5%
Only at night and at naptime 5.1%
Used to, but not anymore...26.3%
Sucks fingers or thumb..7.1%

Does your baby watch TV – either baby developmental DVDs or sports with Daddy?

Never, are you nuts?...7.4%
Occasionally glances at the TV if it's on,
   but I do not encourage it for any length of time...................25.3%
Maybe 30 minutes a day or less 31.6%
One to 3 hours a day..31.6%
TV is always on (baby loves Oprah!) 6.3%

Some additional comments included:
- Only on weekends, movies usually.
- The older kids watch more, the 2½-year-old occasionally watches, the 3½-year-old autistic child has to have it on.
- His older sister watches a lot.
- Didn't watch anything till 2 years old—not big TV watchers.

Playdates

Once a week during a class (other babies have germs!).............7.3%
Twice a week during a class (structured playdates ROCK).........8.5%
Once a week with friends in the park (or home) 25.6%
More than once a week with friends in a casual environment...36.6%
BOTH – can't have enough playdates!!!...............................19.5%
None – who has time for playdates? 11.0%

Additional playdate comments:
- Not during baby's first 3 months.
- He is in school 5 days a week.
- Went to Gymboree or Music Together classes from 6 months to 2 years. Always playdates at a friend's.
- Once a week at Mommy & Me or more if I can schedule playdates.
- We have twins, so they have built-in playdates.
- One to two times a month at a friend's house.
- Monthly is all I have time for!
- At the park daily.

Does your baby...?

Stay home with you or another family member 66.7%
Stay home with a nanny..8.3%
Go to daycare...17.9%
Go to preschool 22.6%

Some additional comments:
- Stays at home on weekends with parents and weekdays at the grandparents' house.
- Three days a week with nanny, 4 days at home with mommy.
- One day a week in daycare.
- Have done all of the above.
- Goes to work with me Monday thru Friday (I'm so lucky!).
- At home half the time, at his father's store the other half of the time.
- Home with me in the mornings—daycare in the afternoons.

When your child was 0-12 months, what did you do when you needed to take a shower or cook? (more than one answer is fine).

Put them in a playpen with toys ....31.2 %

Took my shower during their naptime ....59.1 %

TV time – thank you Baby Einstein and PBS ....16.1 %

Had a neighbor come over for 10 minutes 1.1%

Took them in the shower with me,

   or strapped them to me while cooking 30.1%

Other 33.3%

Other choices:

- Put them in the bouncer. *(This was a popular answer.)*
- Waited for husband.
- I put her in her car seat and brought her in the bathroom with me.
- Older brothers and sisters helped out.
- Skipped shower regularly!
- Put them in the high chair with toys and brought them in the bathroom with me so they weren't alone.

What types of things do you do for YOURSELF as a mom for "me" time (check all that apply).

Yoga 7.3%

Sleep 36.5%

Bath 33.3%

Read..52.1%

Lunch with friends...28.1%

Date night 26.0%

Work out 29.2%

What is me time? Who am I? 34.4%

Additional comments:

- Watch TV or movie.
- Go tanning twice a week.

- As socializing is difficult with autism, and housebound...had to get creative...just now discovering this avenue—Facebook!!
- Jewelry-making, trade shows, pedicure.
- Other spa treatments, like pedicure or massage.
- Three of our four kids have SPD and/or autism spectrum disorder. The youngest two just turned 6 in December, and we are finally able to go out on a date a few times here and there.
- It is rare that I get out without my son, and when I do, I feel guilty most of the time. However, when he is with me, I find myself wishing for time apart.
- Just sit with peace 'n quiet.
- Scrapbook and date night occasionally.
- Blog.

As your toddler turned 3 and 4 years old, did they continue to nap?

Yes, every day 20.5%
Sometimes, less as they got older 40.9%
Never 29.5%
They were too hard to get to sleep at that age 9.1%

Have you ever had your child evaluated by an occupational therapist?

Yes (If yes, please add your child's diagnoses if any) 61.1%
No 38.9%

Diagnoses include:
Pervasive developmental delay—not otherwise specified, sensory issues, autism, global developmental delay, delayed language, anxiety, depression, attention-deficit/hyperactivity disorder, epilepsy, cerebral palsy, Asperger syndrome, learning disability, hearing problems, attachment disorder, spinal muscular atrophy

If your child has special needs, does your child receive any special services?

Occupational therapy..83.1%
Speech therapy..79.9%
Physical therapy...20.3%

If yes, which setting and how often?
- Tri-county provides once a week.
- OT, two times weekly for 30 minutes.
- OT one time a week at home, speech therapy one time a week at the clinic.
- Through IEP at school.
- Speech therapy, 60 minutes per month; OT, 1 hour a week at preschool.
- Once per week for each.

If your child has sensory issues, did they have the following? (skip question if no sensory concerns).

Premature birth—if so, how many weeks?...........................31.7%
Medical issues—please list...43.3%
Ear infections..48.3%
Difficulties with vaccinations—please explain.....................20.0%
Feeding difficulties—please explain................................50.0%

Parents reports:
- She received oxygen the first day of life. She had stomach problems and acid reflux for the first year at least. She was unable to breastfeed. She continues to be a "picky" eater.
- Had a horrible reaction to the MMR vaccination.
- Has dairy allergies.
- Had a reaction to the flu shot with thermisol.
- Could not/would not nurse.
- Has autistic spectrum disorder.

- Has an oral aversion due to being on a ventilator for 3 weeks.
- Was born at 30 weeks.
- Autism onset after MMR vaccinations at 14 months—he has difficulty eating mushy foods (ie, mashed potatoes) or anything green.
- Was born 2 weeks early (just barely "full term"). Induced birth with Pitocin. Extreme colic. No sleep. Excessive spitting up and drooling. Low weight gain. Eczema. Cradle cap. Food allergies. Night terrors. Constipation.
- Jude had to get ear tubes at 13 months because his hearing was 80% blocked.
- My son has neurofibromatosis 1, as well as pervasive developmental disorder—not otherwise specified. He did have minor feeding issues and had to have soy formula.
- Had gastrointestinal issues as an infant, had a milk protein allergy.

Would you consider a variety of therapies for your baby or toddler? You may pick more than one answer.

Never, Western PhDs for my little one ONLY! 2.4%

Yes, GF/CF diet (or any special diet) 52.9%

Yes, music therapy 83.5%

Yes, aromatherapy 42.4%

Yes, auditory integration therapy for little one's ears 52.9%

Yes, acupressure/acupuncture 40.0%

Yes, baby massage (touch therapy) 68.2%

Yes, light therapy..31.8%

Other? Please comment 15.3%

Other therapies:
- Chi Quiong.
- We tried GF/CF and it did not seem to have an effect.
- Anthroposophic medicine finally helped, more than anything.
- Hesitant of acupuncture, but yes, acupressure.
- "Joining play therapy."
- Naturopathic medicine.

- Hippotherapy.
- I would consider any if needed.
- At his age, we've tried everything imaginable...except medical marijuana. It's not legal in our state, but if it were, I think I'd try that. I've read some really promising articles on the subject. *(Grasping at straws at this point, perhaps?)*
- Suggest it! I'm open.
- Craniosacral therapy, intensive behavioral intervention, developmental therapy, psychosocial rehabilitation, feeding therapy group.
- Integrated Listening Therapy; however, all are considered complementary therapies for us; OT is our primary intervention.

What is the one thing about being a parent you wished someone would have told you? Or maybe you were told and didn't listen. Please share.

1. The one thing that I wish I would have done earlier was unstructured play dates. I was so nervous about my son's interactions with other children his own age because of his size, strength, and high pain tolerance that I micromanaged his interactions. I think he missed out on development of some valuable social-interaction skills because of this.

2. I wish someone would have prepared me better for the worry you experience as a parent. It's many times worse than I imagined.

3. No matter the challenges, there is much joy.

4. Well, having an autistic child was not something we planned, but we love him just the same. He is very cool in many ways, despite his disability. I wish I knew what caused it (we think it is genetic). But, it is what it is...I definitely didn't want any more kids, though.

5. I wish someone would have told me that some kids react very negatively to vaccines and that administering them could very well cause autism.

6. I wish I would have known that some kids have adverse reactions to vaccinations and that there was a possibility of autism.

7. There are never any guarantees.

8. So much! I wish I'd cut out dairy and soy when nursing, fed her only organics from the beginning, avoided gluten for the first year, not vaccinated at all, not used a toxic exterminator for our bugs, not gotten my mercury fillings removed while nursing, spent more time outdoors, followed Weston Price nutritional principles from before conception on, never fed her Tylenol or antibiotics, never used those awful topical steroids, sent her to a Waldorf school from the beginning, investigated my own family's and my husband's family's medical risk factors (he had a severe milk allergy as a child and never warned me! And my mother had eczema and never mentioned it!), and just in general I wish I had not wasted so much time and money on useless Western allopathic medical "specialists"—I should have gone to anthroposophist doctors from the beginning.

9. How wonderful it is, even with all that it entails!

10. EASY: Eat, Activity, Sleep, You (mom). This really helped me get Jude on a routine as a baby.

11. Applied behavioral therapy and counseling helped me to better understand and prepare for the worse before it got better...I got more education and training for home-integration use. I made a bad choice thinking it was killing his spirit...acting out behavior became worse. I was afraid that it was causing him to feel "wrong" and demeaned. Ugh! I just didn't understand how the autistic mind worked, then. I am not sure they did either, 10 years ago.

12. Very specific answers for how to deal with problem behavior without corporal punishment.

13. When my mother and sister noticed my child wasn't doing all the things in his developmental stage, I didn't respond to them and I wished I would have listened a little more. I could have gotten him

a better start, but as a parent, we all think our children are perfect little creatures.

14. There's nothing anyone can say, your life completely changes when you become a parent. Love will pour through you, and your heart will break every day over good things, bad things, holding on, and letting go.

15. Parenting changes from child to child and from parent to parent. It's OK for Dad to do things differently, it works and it is a great way for baby and Dad to bond. Just because something works for one person doesn't mean it will work for you.

16. To pick your battles!

17. Do what you feel is right, deep inside, and what works for you. Don't feel pressured by other mothers around you who force-feed you with information about what THEY think you should be doing. EVERY child and EVERY family is different.

18. I was told to put my children to bed and let them cry themselves to sleep. I'm SOOOOOO glad I didn't listen that that advice. I found other ways to teach them to rely on themselves, and they KNOW that I will always be there for them.

19. That you don't have to have a baby to be a mother. This young man is my stepson, but I don't advertise that fact, and not many people realize that. He is my son and I love him as my own.

20. I always thought that parents who scheduled their lives around their kids' naps were hypersensitive hyperschedulers. Now I know it was self-preservation! Getting good, regular naps makes everyone's life better...our social calendar adjusts much easier.

21. Always expect the unexpected, never doubt your instincts, and always believe in your heart that no matter how hard your day is, your child's is usually much, much harder.

22. When your kids are grown with kids of their own, you might be raising them for them.

23. Question doctors, even when they say "everything's fine." When you only have one child and they are delayed, how do you know what is considered 'typical?'

24. Discipline is more work for the parent than for the child. I never understood that!!

25. Relax and enjoy, they grow so fast.

26. Nothing at all.

27. How wonderful it is to have the love of your child and how much you can love your child.

28. It doesn't get easier...just different.

29. That every decision you make about your child somehow ends up making you feel guilty, and too many people feel it is their right to tell you how you are doing as a parent, even when you don't want to know.

30. It is hard!

31. How isolating and sad it is, and how much discrimination we all suffer, not to mention how it affects not only my child but her sister and her family!

32. *** No one ever told me the risk of vaccinations, especially to a child who already has a compromised immune system—one size does not fit all! ***

33. That my child could be born with autism. Maybe then I could have been prepared.

34. To completely trust your gut instinct. Even when your family members, doctors, and/or teachers tell you it's just your child's age, gender, or ambition level. Only you know your child. Advocate, advocate, advocate!!!!

35. How different each child is, and you will never have the answers.

36. I wish someone had told me that having a preemie was not just a NICU thing and to know that it is okay to be concerned about your child even after that. Too many people tried to tell me to relax once my

daughter was out of the NICU. The reality is, we have been on a long journey of helping her. It really hurts when people try to admonish me for being a concerned parent. With the recent autism diagnosis, believe me, the critics have been completely silenced. How sad.

37. How hard it is when your child was struggling and you couldn't find the answers, and no one seemed to want to even listen to the questions...

38. The value of early occupational therapy!!!

39. When we got his diagnosis, I grieved for days. All I could say was, 'this isn't what I wanted for him.' Pregnancy is all about getting ready for a new baby, and that's all anyone wants to give advice about. I wish someone had prepared me for the overwhelming feelings that develop as they get older. That's when you get beyond the baby and start to meet the person they'll become, which makes it infinitely more heartbreaking when they have a problem that will make their entire life harder.

40. That sleep would be a thing of the past. But that it would be worth it.

41. Never underestimate—or overestimate—the support you might get from other parents.

42. To trust my instincts. To be more forceful when I felt doctors, etc, weren't listening to me.

43. I always hoped for a healthy child but never knew that my son could be perfectly healthy yet have a mental disorder. He has autism. I wish someone could've prepared me that being a mother would be such a challenge...but I guess there is no way to really prepare. I always fall back on the incredible love I have for my little boy!

44. It's going to mean sometimes you need to react like a robot to get though to your child. Often removing yourself from what you are feeling for their needs.

45. I don't think it was that I didn't listen as much as I didn't fully comprehend how I would love my child and do anything in my power to help him achieve success.

46. That being a parent is harder than it looks.

47. To have my son evaluated by a neurodevelopmental pediatrician earlier.

48. Try whatever feels right, and if something is not going correctly— do what feels right.

49. They all grow up eventually, so enjoy the moments!

50. I wish I had listened and taken time for me. I also wish that I would let others help me more.

51. Life is like a box of chocolates, many different flavors and variety. One is different from the other, but don't judge.

52. Just the standard, "I knew everything before I became a parent."

53. I misinterpreted the milestones questions. There were quite a few red flags, and the pediatrician I had just did not get it either—even after my son had been diagnosed elsewhere. So we switched pediatricians. My son was fascinated with hair and would try and eat it. Any length of hair—stray hair—he would play with it and eat it. I was so worried about a bezoar in his stomach. He did not pull out his own hair—there was enough of mine around, even though I vacuumed all the time and kept my hair up. He would find and play with an eyelash. I tried teaching him stories/letters and songs, and he would just not seem to care. I did not want to seem pushy. When he was reaching for something he shouldn't, or get into trouble, I would give him the no-no look and he would just give me this blank look like he really did not understand my expression— and I still did not get it. To get him to learn to come to his name, I had to make animal noises. If I was at the other end of the house going potty and heard a funny noise—maybe something falling— I would squeak at him like a guinea pig and he would come running. So I would add in his name. It was quite hilarious being at a La Leche League meeting—looking for him and squeaking like a guinea pig to get him to come to me or find me.

54. Getting an IEP WILL help—even if the classification is under the autism umbrella—keep asking questions of professionals and keep researching—blogs can be great resources. Parent each child as they need to be parented—NOT how YOU want to parent.

55. It is going to be a lot of work. Get sleep when you can, especially for the first few years. Take care of yourself while you are parenting—it is NOT a crime to care for yourself. Be an advocate for your child—there are a lot of great teachers and administrators; however, there are also some who really don't care about your child.

56. Hire help after birth if you can afford it, and sleep. Thinking becomes pretty distorted after a while of sleeping only 1-2 hours at a time.

57. How much more work it is to have two kids.

58. It's both way harder, yet way easier than I'd ever imagined!

59. The worry that you encounter when you have children! I worry about them constantly!

60. To be more aware of the hormonal fluctuations after birth. And that they can come on suddenly months afterwards and possibly continue for up to 18 months.

61. There isn't a lot that I wish someone had told me because I read every single book I could find about babies and toddlers. I read everything and then formed my own parenting philosophy. My only advice to new moms is to not take advice, and educate yourself.

62. I wish someone had told me how to deal with a picky eater. It has been hard in the past to introduce new foods to my 9-year-old.

63. How important a routine was.

64. Keep them in their own beds to sleep at night.

65. Structure is key.

66. I didn't really believe that my second would be completely opposite from my first, when I used the same parenting philosophies, sleep routines, sign language, etc. My first used 25 to 30 signs before she

started talking. This made communication wonderful. My little boy watches us, smiles, and screams at us instead of signing. My first pretty much puts herself down for a nap, and my second cries every time we enter his room because he knows it's naptime. They really are sooooo different, but it's a lot of fun!

67. Shots just wait. You are a mom, and you know best. If your doctor won't listen, find a new one!!!!

68. Sorry, but I am still figuring that one out...

69. That it is the hardest thing to do because it's 24/7. Even more so when there are special needs.

70. Enjoy your sleep now; when you have kids, you don't get much sleep. Sooo true!

Appendix B

Must-Have Baby Kit

AFTER INTERVIEWING SEVERAL MOMS, I ASSEMBLED A LIST OF THE "MUST Haves" you should prepare for when you first bring your baby home:

- Car seat—one with a good safety rating
- Diapers and wipes—try a few different brands out to see what works for you and your baby
- A bath seat for the sink and a soft wash cloth (with organic baby wash)
- Clothes (including Onesies, warm clothes for colder climates, layers so that your baby doesn't get too hot or too cold, cozy and soft materials without tags)
- Mylicon, for baby gas
- Safety nail clippers
- Desitin, Boudreaux's Butt Paste, or some sort of diaper cream
- Breast pump
- Bottles
- Binkies
- Burp cloths
- Boppy pillow for breastfeeding or bottle-feeding
- Swaddling blankets and knowing the technique for swaddling
- Calming womb sounds or music for baby
- A swing or bouncy seat to put the baby down in during the day
- A baby monitor (the video ones seem to be popular lately)

References

1. Cohen LJ. *Playful Parenting: A Bold New Way to Nurture Close Connections, Solve Behavior Problems, and Encourage Children's Confidence.* New York, NY: Ballantine; 2001.

2. Madaule P. *When Listening Comes Alive: A Guide to Effective Learning and Communication.* Norval, Ontario, Canada: Moulin Publishing; 1994:93.

3. Medina J. *Brain Rules: 12 Principles for Surviving and Thriving at Work, Home, and School.* Seattle, WA: Pear Press; 2008:156.

4. Elliot L. *What's Going on in There? How the Brain and Mind Develop in the First Five Years of Life.* USA: Bantam; 1999:38-39.

5. Johnson SR. Teaching Our Childen to Write, Read and Spell—A Developmental Approach. www.youandyourchildshealth.org. Accessed June 4, 2010.

6. Tethered spinal cord syndrome. Wikipedia. http://en.wikipedia.org/wiki/Tethered_spinal_cord_syndrome. Accessed May 27, 2010.

7. Elliot L. *What's Going on in There? How the Brain and Mind Develop in the First Five Years of Life.* USA: Bantam; 1999:205-206.

8. Medina J.*Brain Rules: 12 Principles for Surviving and Thriving at Work, Home, and School.* Seattle, WA: Pear Press; 2008:33-34.

9. Case-Smith J. *Occupational Therapy for Children.* 4th ed. St Louis, MO: Mosby; 2001:85-87.

10. Cohen LJ. *Playful Parenting: A Bold New Way to Nurture Close Connections, Solve Behavior Problems, and Encourage Children's Confidence.* New York, NY: Ballantine; 2001:93-112.

11. Kranowitz C. *The Out-of-Sync Child.* New York, NY: Berkley Publishing Group/ Penguin Books; 2005.

12. Wilbarger P. The Wilbarger Deep Pressure and Proprioceptive Technique and Oral Tactile Technique. www.OT-Innovations.com. Accessed May 31, 2010.

13. Miller LJ. *Sensational Kids: Hope and Help for Children with Sensory Processing Disorder (SPD).* New York, NY: G.P. Putmam's Sons; 2006.

14. Biel L, Peske N. *Raising a Sensory Smart Child: The Definitive Handbook for Helping Your Child with Sensory Processing Issues.* New York, NY: Penguin Books; 2009.

15. Kranowitz C, Newman J. *Growing an In-Sync Child.* New York, NY: The Penguin Group; 2010.

16. Young G. *Essential Oils Integrative Medical Guide.* USA: Essential Science Publishing; 2006:26.

17. McClure VS. *Infant Massage: A Handbook for Loving Parents.* New York, NY: Bantam Books; 2000.

18. Deadman P, Al-Khafaji M, Baker K. A manual of acupuncture. East Sussex: *J Chin Med Publications.* 1998.

19. Challem J. *The Food-Mood Solution.* Hoboken, NJ: John Wiley & Sons; 2007:4.

20. Somer E. *Food & Mood: The Complete Guide to Eating Well and Feeling Your Best.* New York, NY: Holt Paperbacks; 1999:61.

21. Somer E. *Food & Mood: The Complete Guide to Eating Well and Feeling Your Best.* New York, NY: Holt Paperbacks; 1999:46.

22. Challem J. *The Food-Mood Solution.* Hoboken, NJ: John Wiley & Sons; 2007:30.

23. Cordain L. *The Paleo Diet: Lose Weight and Get Healthy by Eating the Foods You Were Designed to Eat.* Hoboken, NJ: John Wiley & Sons; 2002:86-87.

24. Challem J. *The Food-Mood Solution.* Hoboken, NJ: John Wiley & Sons; 2007:52.

25. Bock K. *Healing the New Childhood Epidemics Autism, ADHD, Asthma, and Allergies.* New York, NY: Ballantine Books; 2008:204-205.

26. Case-Smith J. *Occupational Therapy for Children.* 4th ed. St Louis, MO: Mosby; 2001:85-87, 528-535.

27. Case-Smith J. *Occupational Therapy for Children.* 4th ed. St Louis, MO: Mosby; 2001:163-164.

28. Case-Smith J. *Occupational Therapy for Children.* 4th ed. St Louis, MO: Mosby; 2001:155-156.

29. Case-Smith J. *Occupational Therapy for Children.* 4th ed. St Louis, MO: Mosby; 2001:163-164.

Resources

Sᴇɴsᴏʀʏ Wᴏʀʟᴅ, ᴀ ᴘʀᴏᴜᴅ ᴅɪᴠɪsɪᴏɴ ᴏꜰ Fᴜᴛᴜʀᴇ Hᴏʀɪᴢᴏɴs, ɪs ᴛʜᴇ ᴡᴏʀʟᴅ's largest publisher devoted exclusively to resources for those interested in sensory processing disorder. They also sponsor national conferences for parents, teachers, therapists, and others interested in supporting those with sensory processing disorder. Visit *www.sensoryworld.com* for further information.

Sᴇɴsᴏʀʏ Wᴏʀʟᴅ

721 W Abram St

Arlington, TX 76013

Phone: (800) 489-0727 or (817) 277-0727

Fax: (817) 277-2270

info@sensoryworld.com

www.sensoryworld.com

Sensory products include *Answers to Questions Teachers Ask about Sensory Intgration, The Goodenoughs Get in Sync, The Sensory Connection, Prechool SENSE, Starting SI Therapy, MoveAbout Cards, 28 Instant Songames, Songames for Sensory Integration, Danceland, Marvelous Mouth Music, The Out-of-Sync Child* video, *Making Sense of Sensory Integration, Teachers Ask about Sensory Integration, Seeing Clearly,* and *Soothing the Senses.*

Web Sites

American Academy of Pediatrics
www.aap.org

Information about auditory integration therapy
www.ait1st.com

American Occupational Therapy Association
www.aota.org

Dr Sears' Web site for general baby questions
www.askdrsears.com

www.babies-and-sign-language.com

Future Horizons
www.fhautism.com

Occupational therapy equipment and developmental toys
www.Funandfunction.com

Registered dietician Julie Matthews,
who specializes in diets for children with autism
www.healthfulliving.org

Information on music therapy
www.integrativemusictherapyla.com

Parenting with Love and Logic
www.loveandlogic.com

A comprehensive Web site with tons of gluten-free,
casien-free, soy-free, and more foods that you can order
for anyone with food sensitivities
www.nulifefoods.com

Our Web site
www.sensoryparenting.com

www.SensorySmarts.com

www.signingbaby.com

Information about sensory processing disorder
www.SPDfoundation.net

Our nonprofit organization
www.SpecialNeedsUnited.org

Occupational therapy DVDs
www.TRPWellness.com

www.webmd.com

Zaky and the Kangaroo Zak available at *www.zakeez.com*

RESOURCES

Books

Aromatherapy for the Healthy Child, by Valarie Ann Worwood

The Baby Book, by William Sears, MD, and Martha Sears, RN

The Baby Whisperer Solves All Your Problems, by Tracy Hogg and Melinda Blau

Brain Rules, by John Medina

Essential Oils Integrative Medical Guide, by D. Gary Young, ND

Growing an In-Sync Child: Simple, Fun Activities to Help Every Child Develop, Learn and Grow, by Carol Kranowitz, MA, and Joyce Newman, MA

The Happiest Baby on the Block: The New Way to Calm Crying and Help Your Newborn Sleep Longer, by Harvey Karp

How to Grow Fresh Air: 50 Houseplants That Purify Your Home or Office, by B. C. Wolverton

Just Take a Bite: Easy, Effective Answers to Food Aversions and Eating Challenges, by Lori Ernsperger, PhD, and Tania Stegen-Hanson, OTR/L

Nobody Ever Told Me (Or My Mother) That! Everything from Bottles and Breathing to Healthy Speech Development, by Diane Bahr, MS, CCC-SLP

The Out-of-Sync Child Has Fun, by Carol Kranowitz—this book provides fun activities for you and your child

Parenting a Child with Sensory Processing Disorder: A Family Guide to Understanding and Supporting Your Sensory-Sensitive Child, by Christopher R. Auer, MA, with Susan Blumberg, PhD

Playful Parenting, by Lawrence J. Cohen, PhD

Raising a Sensory Smart Child: The Definitive Handbook for Helping Your Child with Sensory Processing Issues, by Lindsey Biel and Nancy Peske

Sensational Kids: Hope and Help for Children with Sensory Processing Disorder, by Dr Lucy Jane Miller and Doris Fuller

Sensitive Sam: Sam's Sensory Adventure Has a Happy Ending! by Marla Roth-Fisch (for kids!)

Touching; The Human Significance of Skin, by Ashley Monagu

The Vaccine Book: Making the Right Decision for Your Child,
  by Robert W. Sears, MD, FAAP

Vaccine Safety Manual: for Concerned Families and Health Practioners,
  by Neil Miller

Index

A

Acupressure/acupuncture, 248–50, 294
Addictions, 259
ADHD (attention-deficit/hyperactivity
    disorder), 223–24
Adrenaline, 262
Air fresheners, 12, 24
Airplanes, 34–35, 183–84
Allergies, 24, 133–34, 256, 264–67
Anger, 132, 140
Animals
    outdoor, 121
    pets, 115–21
    stuffed, 73
Applied Behavioral Analysis (ABA), 170
Arcades, 172–73
Aromatherapy, 234–36, 294
Aspiration, 283
Asymmetrical tonic neck reflex, 50
Auditory development, 81
Auditory integration therapy, 242–46, 294
Auditory processing disorder, 224–25
Autism, 118, 215–22, 237, 240
Ayres, A. Jean, 209

B

Baby
    body clock of, 45
    bonding with, 19–25, 39, 274
    changing, 12–13, 26–28
    dressing, 28–30
    feeding, 35–41
    holding, 23
    premature, 271–77
    preparing for, 1–16
    transporting, 31–35
    uniqueness of, 2
Baby Bumblebee DVDs, 64
Baby Einstein DVDs, 65
Baby food, 261
Baby kit, must-have, 303
Baby massage, 246–47, 294
Baby-proofing, 14–15, 79
Babysitters, 104–5, 123–24
Balls, 32–33, 94
Basketball, 195
Bathing, 25–26, 94, 125, 155–56
Bathrooms
    cleaning, 254
    organizing, 13
Beach outings, 173–74
Beads, 193
Beanbags, 94
Bedding, 8, 10, 255
Bedrooms, 11
Bed-wetting, 151–52
Behavioral issues, 134–35, 167–71, 206–7
Berard AIT, 242–46
Biel, Lindsey, 210
Binkies. *See* Pacifiers
Birds, 116
Blankets, security, 91
Blocks, 73, 86, 95, 195
Blogs, 125
Body carriers, 33
Bonding, 19–25, 39, 129–30, 274
Books, 54, 73, 86, 94
Bottle-feeding, 35, 38–41, 289
Breastfeeding, 35–39, 41, 128, 289
Broca area, 237

Brushing techniques, therapeutic, 205–6
Bubbles, 94
Buses, 34–35
By Kids Only, 72

C

Caffeine, 262
Calvanese, Emily, 248–50
Candles, 12, 24
Carpets, cleaning, 253–54
Carriers, 31–33
Cars, 8, 33–34, 183
Cats, 116
Cerebral palsy, 282
Chickens, 121
Choices, giving, 142–44
Churches, 174
Cigarettes, 25
Cleaning products, 25, 253–55
Clothing, 28–30, 157, 255
Clutter, 13–14
Coloring, 93
Communication, 138–42.
    See also Language; Speech
    and language development
Cooperative interaction, 185
Cortisol, 246, 262
Cosmetics, 252–53
Cravings, 259
Crawling, 51, 61–62
Crayons, 93
Cruising, 77–78

D

Daycare, 110–13, 290
Dental care, 154, 174–75, 253
Dentists, 192
Developmental milestones
    0 to 6 months, 55–58
    6 to 12 months, 74–76
    1 to 2 years, 96–102
    2 to 3 years, 197–200
    concerns about, 101–2
    premature babies and, 272
Diaper rash, 27
Diapers. See also Potty training
    changing, 12–13, 26–28
    cloth vs disposable, 28

Diet. See also Feeding; Food
    effects of, 257–58
    protein in, 262–63
    salt in, 263
    sugar in, 263–64
Discipline, 167–71
Disneyland, 182
Doctors, 174–75, 192
Dogs, 117–18
Dressing, 28–30, 157
Dunn, Winnie, 211
DVDs, 64–66, 123

E

Ear infections, 21, 34, 82–83
Easels, 193
Elimination diet, 264, 267
Epilepsy, 284
Essential oils. See Aromatherapy
Exercise balls, 32–33
Exhaustion, 137

F

Facebook, 125
Falling, 77–78
Family members, 113–14, 123–24
Farmers' markets, 175–76
Feeding. See also Diet; Food
    bottle-, 35, 38–41, 289
    breast-, 35–39, 41, 289
    issues, 228–32
    station, 12
Ferrets, 118
Fish, 119
Floppy babies, 283
Food. See also Diet; Feeding
    addiction and, 259
    allergies, 133, 264–67
    baby, 261
    intolerances, 133–34, 267–69
    introducing new, 88, 228–32
    marketing campaigns for, 260
    monitoring reactions to, 260
    mood and, 258
    organic, 261
    relationship with, 259
    sensory nature of, 258–59
Football, 195

INDEX

Fruits, 261–62
Fun and Function, 72
Furniture, 9–10

G

GABA (gamma-aminobutyric acid), 262
Gak, 195–96
Gerbils, 119–20
"Good-bye," saying, 161–62
Gravitational insecurity, 32
Grocery stores, 176–77
Gross- and fine-motor development
    0 to 6 months, 55–57
    6 to 12 months, 74–76
    1 to 2 years, 84–85, 96–100
    2 to 3 years, 197–99
Guinea pigs, 119–20
Gymboree, 67–68

H

Haircuts, 152–53
Hair spray, 252
Hamsters, 119–20
Hands, washing, 156–57
Health Master, 232
Hearing, sense of, xx, 20–21, 81.
    See also Auditory development;
    Auditory processing disorder
Heller, Sharon, 211
"Hello," saying, 161–62
Help, seeking, 225–26
Herwill-Levin, Khymberleigh, 242–46
Home
    baby-proofing, 14–15
    organizing, 11–16
Hooked on Phonics, 66
Hospital stays, 277–81
House, playing, 191
Humor, sense of, 132
Hunger, 135
Hypersensitivity, 201–4
Hyposensitivity, 201–4
Hypotonia, 283

I

Insulin, 135
Integrative Music Therapy, 240–241
Internet, conducting research on, 283

J

Juicers, 231–32
Jumping, 193–94

K

Kangaroo Zak, 275–76
Kitchen
    cleaning, 254
    organizing, 13
    pretend, 191

L

Lactose intolerance, 88, 267
Language. *See also* Speech and language
    development
    second, 65–66
    sign, 65, 69–70
Laundry, 254–55
Lee, Andrea, 218–22
Libraries, 177
Lighting, 11–12
Light therapy, 233–34, 294
Little Pim DVDs, 65
Living room, 11–12
Lizards, 120–21
Lovey, favorite, 91

M

Malls, 177
Massage, 246–47, 294
Mattresses, 10
Memory, 5
Mental retardation, 283–84
"Me" time, 128–29, 291–92
Milk, 260, 264, 267–68
Miller, Lucy Jane, 201, 204, 210
Mind, changing, 144
Mirroring, 20, 52
Mirrors, 54
Mobiles, 3, 53

Mold, 255–56
Mommy & Me, 68
Moods, 258
Moon Sand, 195–96
Motion sickness, 34, 183–84
Movies, 178
Museums, 178
Music, 5–8
Musical instruments, 73, 194–95
Musick, Shanna, 80–81
Music therapy, 236–42, 294

N

Nail polish, 252
Nails, trimming, 154–55
Nannies, 105–10, 290
Naps, 47–48, 92, 158, 292
Night-lights, 234
Noise, 4–7
Nose, blowing, 153
NuLife Foods, 269
Nursery
    auditory considerations for, 4–8
    bedding for, 8, 10
    decorating, 3
    furniture for, 9–10
    painting, 3
    tactile considerations for, 8

O

OBOZ (On Behalf of Zachary) program,
    276
Obstacle courses, 196
Occupational therapy
    definition of, 207
    determining need for, 58
    sensory integration and, 207–9
    survey results on, 292–93
Oral aversions, 228–31
Oral-motor skills, 227–28
Oral stimulation, 229–31
Organic food, 261
Outings, 172–85

P

Pacifiers, 24, 41, 159–60, 289
Paints, 3, 193
"Parenting with Love and Logic"
    approach, 169–70
Parents
    acupressure for, 250
    humor and, 132
    role of, in play, 186–89
    sleep for, 48–49, 92
    stay-at-home, 122–25
    thick skin for, 132
    working, 126–30
Parks, 179
Pasta jewelry, 193
Peek-a-boo, 20, 52
Pets, 115–21
Physical therapy, 293
Picky eaters, 228–32
Plants, 255
Play. See also Toys
    0 to 6 months, 51–53
    6 to 12 months, 70–72
    1 to 2 years, 92–93
    2 to 3 years, 185–92
    frequency of, 70–71
    importance of, 51
    location for, 15–16, 51–52
    overstimulation and, 52–53
    role of parents in, 186, 187–89
    rules and, 187
    social, 93
    types of, 71, 185
Playdates, 163–65, 290
Play-Doh, 195–96
Playgrounds, indoor, 68–69
Playgroups, structured, 67–68
Plumbing, 13
Potty training, 144–52
Preemies, 271–77
Pregnancy, length of, 288
Pretend play, 190
Proprioceptive sense, xx, 22, 89–90
Protein, 262–63
Public transportation, 34–35
Pumping, 128
Puzzles, 73, 86, 94, 193
PVC (polyvinyl chloride), 9–10

Q

Quiet time, 141–42

R

Rabbits, 120
Rats, 120
Rattles, 52–54
Reaching, 61
Reading, 66–67, 73
Redirecting, 170–71
Refuge, sensory, 115
Reptiles, 120–21
Restaurants, 180
Riding toys, 95
Rocking chairs, 9
Rolling over, 59–60
Roughhousing, 189–90
Rugs, cleaning, 253–54

S

Safety, 14–15, 79, 187
Salt, 263
School, playing, 192
Screaming, 140
Seasickness, 184
Seizures, 284
Self-soothing, 90–91
Sensory integration, xx, 207–8
Sensory integration dysfunction.
        See Sensory processing disorder
Sensory issues
    addressing, 206–7
    allergies vs, 133–34
    awareness of, 133, 288
    behavioral vs, 134–35, 206–7
    eating and, 258–59
    exhaustion vs, 137
    with hospital stays, 277–81
    hunger vs, 135
    with potty training, 147, 150–51
    for premature babies, 274–75
    separation anxiety vs, 136
    signs of, 52
    stubbornness vs, 136–37
    survey results on, 288, 293–94
Sensory processing disorder (SPD)
    effects of, 209–10

frequency of, 210
history of, 209
resources for, 210–11
signs of, 211–13
therapy equipment for, 71–72
Sensory seekers and cravers, 204–5
Separation anxiety, 104, 136
Serotonin, 259, 262
Service dogs, 118
Shampoos, 253
Sharing, 164–65
Shoes, 79–81
Shopping centers, 177
Shouting, 140
Siblings, 113–14
SIDS (Sudden Infant Death Syndrome),
        48, 159
Sight, xix–xx, 20. *See also* Visual
        development
Sign language, 65, 69–70
Silent treatment, 141–42
Singing, 21
Sitting, 60–61
Skype, 110
Sleep, baby's
    body clock and, 45
    cues for, 44–45
    expectations for, 42–43
    length of, 288
    location for, 46, 91–92
    methods, 45
    naps, 47–48, 92
    patterns, 46–47
    position for, 48
    schedules for, 43–44, 90
    sensory needs and, 45–46
Sleep, parents', 48–49, 92
Sleep, toddler's
    bedtime routine, 160–61
    location for, 159
    naps, 158, 292
    waking up from, 161
Slides, 194
Smell, sense of. *See also* Aromatherapy
    development of, 55, 86–87
    emotions and, 235–36
    overview of, xx
    sensitivity of, 24–25
Smoking, 25

Snakes, 121
Soaps, 253
Soccer, 195
Social/cognitive development
  0 to 6 months, 56–58
  6 to 12 months, 74–76
  1 to 2 years, 96–99, 101
  2 to 3 years, 161–65, 197–200
  activities for, 64–69
Sound
  bonding and, 20–21
  overview of, xx
  sensitivity to, 4–5
Soy allergies, 264
Spanking, 167
Speech and language development.
    See also Language
  0 to 6 months, 55–58
  6 to 12 months, 74–76
  1 to 2 years, 96–101
  2 to 3 years, 197–199
  ear infections and, 83
Speech therapy, 293
Sports, 195
Stay-at-home moms (and dads), 122–25
"Stop," saying, 139–40
Straws, 232
Stubbornness, 136–37
Sucking, 23–24, 41, 160, 227–28
Sugar, 135, 263–64
Sunscreen, 173–74, 253
Supplements, 232
Survey results, 287–302
Swaddling, 22, 30–31
Swallowing, 41
Swings, 35, 194
Sylvester, Emily, 213–14

T

Talcum powder, 253
Talking, 20–21
Tantrums, 134–36, 141, 165–67
Taste
  development of, 88
  exploring through, 23
  overview of, xix
Technology, 62–67
Teeth, brushing, 154

Teething, 42, 54, 73, 90
Television, 63–64
Theme parks, 180–82
Thumb-sucking, 24, 289
Time-outs, 168
Toddlers
  naps for, 292
Toe-walking, 80–81
Toiletries, 252–53
Tool kits, pretend, 194
Touch
  bonding and, 22–23, 274
  development of, 55, 88–89
  overview of, xix
Touch therapy. *See* Baby massage
Toxins, 251–57
Tox Town, 256–57
Toys. *See also* Play; *individual toys*
  0 to 6 months, 53–54
  6 to 12 months, 70, 73–74
  1 to 2 years, 93–95
  2 to 3 years, 193–96
  received as gifts, 15–16
  sharing, 164–65
Trains, 34–35, 184
Trampolines, 193–94
Travel, 33–35, 183–84
Travel pillows, 12
Tubman, Andy, 236–42
Tummy time, 49–51
Tunnels, 194
Turkeys, 121
Turtles, 121
TV-watching, 289
Tylenol, 17

U

U-Sing, 241

V

Vaccines, 16–17
Vegetables, 261
Vestibular sense
  development of, 83–84
  overview of, xx, 22–23
  poor, 32
Visual development
  0 to 6 months, 55–56

INDEX

6 to 12 months, 74
1 to 2 years, 85–86, 96, 98–100
2 to 3 years, 197–99
Vitamins, 232

W

Walking, 77–81
Washing machines, 254–55
Water, testing, 255
Weiss, Aviva, 70–72
White noise, 6–7
Wilbarger brushing protocol, 205–6
Womb-sound bears, 4–5
Work, 126–30
Wrestling, 189–90

Y

Yelling, 140
Yoga, 68

Z

Zaky, 275–76
Zoos, 184–85

About the Authors

BRITT COLLINS, MS, OTR/L, GRADUATED FROM COLORADO STATE UNIVER-
sity with a masters in occupational therapy and has been practicing in
a variety of settings, including sensory-integration clinics, schools,
homes, rehabilitation facilities, and hospitals. Jackie Linder Olson is a
producer and writer, whose son has SPD.

Jackie and Britt created an occupational-therapy DVD series for parents, caregivers, and educators to teach the basics of occupational
therapy and how it could be implemented in their children's daily lives.
Their DVDs include "OT in the Home," "OT in the School," "OT for Children with Autism, Special Needs and Typical," and "Yoga for Children
with Special Needs."

The duo cofounded Special Needs United, with the goal of introducing occupational therapy to families of children with special needs. Britt
currently resides in Salem, Oregon, and works at Salem Hospital
Regional Rehabilitation Center, a part of Salem Health in the Outpatient
Neuromuscular Department. Jackie resides in Los Angeles, California.
Both can be found touring the country, speaking about the benefits of
occupational therapy for children.